Hunza
Health Secrets
for long life and
happiness

Hunza Health Secrets
for long life and happiness

Renée Taylor

Keats Publishing, Inc. New Canaan, Connecticut

Because I have confidence in the power of truth and of the spirit, I believe in the future of mankind.

DR. ALBERT SCHWEITZER

Acknowledgments

I wish to express my appreciation and gratitude to those who helped me accomplish my goal—the opportunity to share the message of Hunza through this book and lectures around the country with my film HUNZA. . . . THE VALLEY OF ETERNAL YOUTH. Without them the expedition could never have been possible.

First of all I am deeply indebted to Art Linkletter, the famous star of television and radio—the godfather of my Hunza project—for being responsible for fulfilling my dream! He sent Dr. Allen E. Banik to Hunza in 1958, featuring his trip on the People Are Funny and House Party shows. Upon his return I co-authored the book *Hunza Land* to which Mr. Linkletter wrote the introduction.

To the President of Pakistan, Field Marshal Mohammad Ayub Khan, for letting me visit Hunza. And to the government officials for their efficiency and courtesy.

To His Highness, the Mir Mohammed, O.H.D. Jamal Khan, the ruler of Hunza, the Rani and the whole royal family, my thanks for their understanding and generous hospitality. I could never forget my visit to Hunza and my stay in their beautiful palace. Their kindness and friendly attitude will live forever in my memories.

And to the people of Hunza for their willingness to extend a helping hand in moments of danger.

To Mr. Mulford J. Nobbs, president of Whitehorn Publishing Company, Inc., publishers of my first book on Hunza, and Mrs. Nobbs, I am deeply obliged for financially supporting the film project on Hunza, and for their personal friendship.

And to Zygmunt Sulistrowski I bow for making such a superb motion picture, *Hunza. . . . The Valley of Eternal Youth*, which

I have been showing all over the country and abroad, during my lectures.

To Wayne Mitchel, our cameraman, for his assistance and cooperation and to Mr. Agha, a film director of the government of Pakistan for standing by in emergency.

To Joan Cline for her capable assistance with the research work.

To Ruth Boyd Merritt for her patience and tolerance in typing and retyping the manuscript.

For all the travel arrangements and accommodations, my thanks go to the BOAC (British Overseas Airlines Company), and P.I.A (Pakistan International Airlines), for being most cooperative throughout the whole trip around the world. And my special gratitude goes to the Pakistani pilots who so skillfully manoeuvered the little DC-3 from Rawalpindi through the narrow gorge to Gilgit. Indeed, I must praise them, for getting my expedition safely to my destination.

And to many other dedicated men and women whose names I am not mentioning here, but who truly practice the same principles, and who inspired me and gave me courage to undertake that difficult journey, I am indeed grateful to all of you.

Preface

      This book tells the story of Hunza and the Hunza people—people who in over two thousand years of almost complete isolation seem to have evolved a way of living, eating and thinking that has substantially lengthened their lifespan and dramatically reduced susceptibility to most of the illnesses to which "civilized" people are prone.

      Formerly, Hunza was an independent kingdom and a land of mystery; today it is a part of West Pakistan, functioning as an independent state with a king on the throne. One of the smallest monarchies in the world, the whole country is only 100 miles long and in areas scarcely a mile wide.

      The stories told by the few doctors and scientists who were privileged to visit Hunza in the last sixty years have pictured a Garden of Eden, a paradise on earth. The people of Hunza and their secrets of youth and health have become a living legend to the rest of the world.

      In Hunza, people manage to live to over one hundred years of age in perfect mental and physical health; and men father children at ninety. But their greatest achievement is the fact that sickness is rare, that cancer, heart disease, heart attacks, high or low blood pressure and childhood diseases are virtually unknown. There is no juvenile delinquency in Hunza, and divorce is a rarity. There are no jails, police or army, and there is no need for them, as there hasn't been a crime reported for the last one hundred and thirty years.

      Most probably, these same people stirred the imagination of James Hilton when he wrote *Lost Horizon*. People began hoping for eternal life and a new name was born—a name that symbolizes everyone's deep-felt wish for a healthy, happy and long life—Shangri-la!

While the rest of the civilized world talks of nuclear destruction and fallout shelters, the people of this remote state of Pakistan live in peace, harmony and brotherly love. Fear, hatred and jealousy do not exist. They are friendly, hospitable and religious people.

Their king, Mir Mohammed Jamal Khan, is a democratic ruler, loved and respected by his people. He doesn't need any guards or police. The gates of his palace are open to everyone. Due to its geographical location, bordering with Afghanistan, Russia, China, Kashmir and India, with two famous historical passes, Kilik to Russia and Mintaka to China, only a few miles apart, Hunza makes a strategic target. Nevertheless, the Mir of Hunza manages to remain aloof from the fears and troubles of all of them.

What is restricted is the entry of visitors. The reasons are obvious: the trip is very dangerous. First you have to fly practically through the mountains—a narrow gorge serves as the air route to Gilgit, and a slight change in weather to the north ends in disaster. If you are fortunate to reach Gilgit, which is the last stop of modern transportation, from then on you are on your own. You travel on mule or foot or by jeep—if you are lucky to get through before the road is washed out or destroyed by an avalanche, which is practically a daily occurrence. Then you travel over the same mountain passes, treacherous and zigzagging along a fast torrent of icy water which Marco Polo sailed in 1269 coming from Cathay on his way to India.

No travel agency could very well encourage tourists to visit Hunza. In fact, I wonder how many are even aware of its existence. A special-entry permit is required to visit the little paradise, and only a fortunate few have ever obtained the necessary documents. An invitation of the Mir of Hunza is essential, but still the formalities of red tape complicate the matter and practically the president of Pakistan himself has to sanction such a venture.

Secondly, if you are lucky to get there in one piece, there are no hotels, no restaurants and no stores to buy food. You either have to be the guest of the Mir and accept his hospitality, or be a great adventurer and live outdoors and eat out of your own imported can foods.

There have been many tales about the origin of Hunza. One wonders how these people of a Caucasian race found their domicile in these high mountains—the only white-skinned people among the many races of Hindus and Moslems, all of whom are brown-skinned. And what about the derivation of their language, which doesn't resemble any other known tongue in that area? We accept the story that the Hunzakuts are descendants of a few Greek soldiers who deserted the marauding army of Alexander the Great in search of freedom. These soldiers and their Persian wives wandered in search of a home where they could lead a peaceful life. Eventually they found the valley of what is now known as Hunza.

Soon they discovered that nearby was the route from Sinkiang to Kashmir, used by the Chinese traders to carry their valuable goods, so they resumed the life they led in the army. The settlers began to raid the caravans. It was easy. They would throw heavy boulders down on the innocent traders, pushing them into the chasms, then they would recover the loot. The peace of the Himalayas was disturbed by a handful of bandits. Their retreat served as an impregnable fortress—not even an army could conquer them. Genghis Khan tried and so did the English. For many centuries terror lay in these mountains. Some of the old men tell the gruesome stories of their ancestors to their children—as we tell our gruesome fairy tales!

Today the people of Hunza have a wonderful disposition, good health and long life. They are people who are thoroughly convinced that only through unity can they prosper. However, even in the old days their soil and food took priority over fighting. At the time of planting or harvest, no one could tear them away from their duties. And it is true that their strength and endurance were always superior to many neighboring states. They were always avid agriculturists.

Telling their story, one cannot help but admire the great inner strength which enabled these people to change from warlike creatures to peaceful human beings. The mind and body must be made pure before it can be directed to higher things. This cannot be bought cheaply—it must come from within. Perhaps one who has it is not conscious of it, but then the tranquility, once we have it, cannot be lost. And this is why the Hunzakuts were able to conquer anger, hatred, feverish greed and dangerous ambition and establish a perfect balance of body, mind and spirit. Such men can be regarded with reverence. There is a relation between physical, moral and spiritual. Full control is only obvious in a man whose spiritual consciousness is fully realized. A man filled with criminal intent is suddenly hypnotized by the beauty, love and serenity of peace and can forget his evil nature. Using his consciousness, he can coordinate the power of body, mind and soul and become a complete master of himself. Nothing can thwart him. Otherwise, how can you explain such a miraculous change in a group of people who lived a wild life for centuries?

Love is an inherent power that will transform every disharmony. This feeling of love and inner peace keeps the Hunza people looking and remaining young. Love is an innate quality in man and it need only be called forth in order to express all its radiance. Love makes our life smooth, beautiful and healthy and changes our discontent into harmony and happiness. If one has a kind, unselfish, understanding nature, it will show in his eyes and face, in fact in all his features, and give him a radiance coming from the inner glow of love. Divine love is the magnet that draws all good to you.

I bring the message of health, happiness, peace and love from the land of Hunza.

R. T.

Contents

CONTENTS

I.

Journey
Through
the Himalayas

It was just before dawn at the Rawalpindi airport in Pakistan. We were six: Mr. and Mrs. Mulford J. Nobbs, publishers; Zygmunt Sulistrowski, director-producer; Wayne Mitchell, cameraman; Dr. James B. Jones, philosopher, and myself.

We had come a long way, almost 15,000 miles. Hong Kong, Tokyo, Hawaii, Los Angeles and the vastness of the Pacific lay behind us. Ahead, the fabled land where the life expectancy of the average man was well over one hundred years, where there was no disease, no crime, and where the thirst for war was nonexistent.

We were to film a motion picture in the living Shangri-la—Hunza—and, ultimately, to find out just what it was that made the Hunzakuts different from other peoples on earth.

There was only one small building at the edge of the large field, where the plane, a DC 3, was standing, small and lonely in the early morning light, waiting to take us to the Pakistan village of Gilgit. It seemed pitifully small in comparison with the huge jets that had brought us halfway around the world. There was an early-morning stillness.

As the first light of day spread over the horizon, I could see there wasn't a cloud in the sky. The plane would take off. Any indication of unfavorable weather would have been sufficient reason to cancel the flight. To reach Gilgit, the plane has to fly through gorges so narrow that it is impossible to turn around. Once the flight is under way it must be completed. Since planes cannot fly over the Himalayan ranges, pilots must spread their way through the passes which cut between these towering peaks. Low-hanging clouds would obscure vision and disaster could come in a matter of seconds.

The porters transferred our luggage to the plane, lashing it down in the center of the cabin with heavy ropes. After the huge mass was securely tied down, a protective net was thrown over it. I was reminded of some monstrous leather and metal animal that had just been captured. In the small space left on either side of the cargo, seats were attached to the floor of the plane for the passengers. We were traveling in style.

These small DC 3's flying from Rawalpindi to Gilgit are practically the only means of communicating with a very primitive area, and consequently they are rigged primarily for transporting freight. Passengers come as an afterthought. First, cargo is loaded on the plane, and then, if weight and space limitations permit, passengers are taken. On an average flight you might have as a fellow traveler anything from an air compressor to a small tractor.

But that morning there was enough room left to take on quite a few 5-gallon tins of gasoline. It was somewhat disconcerting to know that we were making such a hazardous flight along with several hundred gallons of high-octane gasoline.

The takeoff was wonderful, the little plane soared up into the air like a bird. The flight from Rawalpindi to Gilgit, a distance of 375 miles, is the most spectacular regularly scheduled flight in the world. And at the same time it is the most dangerous.

After leaving Rawalpindi, the plane seemed to head right into the mountains. Then it felt as though we were flying *through* them. The pilot banked and turned the plane with only a few hundred feet to spare through a maze of jagged corridors, sheer walls of stone rising on either side of us to snowcapped peaks above. This was really "flying by the seat of the pants." I suddenly realized how important flight weather conditions can be. The thought of running into clouds sent a cold chill through me.

Although the cabin was not pressurized, we were not aware of the rarefied atmosphere; we were too busy enjoying the wildly beautiful scenery that surrounded us. The two pilots handled their plane with an amazing skill.

Once when the wings seemed only a few feet away from the coarse rock walls of the canyons, I stiffened and gasped in terror.

"Don't worry," someone said, "they've been making this flight for fifteen years and there has been hardly an accident!!" Suddenly the plane banked sharply. I held my breath. *Hardly* gave me little consolation.

Through the small windows we watched the desolate mountains pass by us and below us. We saw mountains and more mountains— the Himalayan magnitude. Mount Nanga Parbat, 26,600 feet high, and its sister peaks soared upward in craggy symmetry. The rough spread of red and brown stone, overlayed with patterns of pristine white snow, sparkled in the brilliance of the sun like a majestic carpet. We could see no roads or foot passes, just wilderness. Far below in some places we caught a glimpse of the timberline, the green of the trees contrasting with the frothy lace of watery torrents from the melting glaciers.

As I sat in the plane, shivering from the cold of the high altitude and shuddering from the fear that we might crash, I tried to think only of the destination of our long journey. The purpose of my trip was to study and photograph the way of life in the Himalayan Shangri-la, the land of Hunza. I was convinced that the true story of Hunza was an illuminating, inspirational message desperately needed by the rest of the world.

I had heard of the physical vigor and the long lives of these people in Hunza: of men and women who were strong and active at over one hundred years of age, in a state of perfect mental and physical health. There were reports of men who had fathered children at the age of ninety, of women who at the age of eighty looked like Western women of forty. Other stories told how there was no cancer, no heart attacks, no vascular complaints—no disease to cut down men and women in the prime of life.

Reports from this earthly paradise were so incredible that they had created worldwide fascination. It didn't seem possible that in this modern age of atomic threats a group of people were living in complete peace, free of the major fears of mankind—disease and war. If the truth about these people could be known, it might help change our pattern of living to one that would promote peace of mind, a healthy body and a longer life.

Below us the character of the terrain began to change. Small farmhouses could be seen dotting the landscape. The mountains seemed to rise directly from the narrow ledges. The plane began to lose altitude, carefully gliding down. As the wheels touched the ground, the plane bounced several times on the rough, dusty airstrip. Then we came to a standstill. Gilgit! We had made it.

It was like stepping into an oven. There was not the slightest movement of air, and the sun beat down on us unmercifully. The temperature was a sizzling 100 degrees.

This was our last contact with modern civilization. I watched the plane wing away over the sun-scorched mountains, not without misgivings. For the next, and final, phase of the trip would be made both by jeep and on foot. Sixty-eight miles away, at the end of a long, arduous and twisting road, lay our final destination: Baltit, the capital of Hunza.

Amid the teeming mass of people who had come to watch the landing was Habibur Rehman Khan, the political agent of Gilgit.

Gilgit is governed by a political agent who serves in the capacity of a governor, judge, policeman and friend. Since Gilgit occupies a position of strategic importance in this remote corner of the world, being only a few miles from the borders of many restless countries, this area is the most important hinterland of Asia.

Along with permits to visit Hunza, permission to pass through Gilgit is necessary. The political agent carefully checks on all visitors and maintains a strict border patrol. He is the law in this Himalayan region.

Every village in Pakistan has a guesthouse provided by the government for the use of visiting military and political personnel. We were invited to stay there, and Mr. Rehman Khan placed his jeep and driver at our disposal. However, when we arrived we found there was scarcely space for a party of six in the two small rooms. Zygmunt, Wayne and Dr. Jones took one room, while the Nobbses and I shared another. The rooms were small, austere and sparsely furnished, but clean. We were crowded, but by now Asian stoicism was beginning to rub off. "Be happy to have a mattress!" Wayne philosophized. He was right.

The food served in the clean dining room looked appetizing and everyone assured me it was very tasty. Nevertheless, while the others ate heartily of the hot, spicy food, I refrained, except for the fresh apricots, which were delicious and straight from the apricot orchard surrounding the guesthouse.

Anxious to see the village, I strolled up the hill to the political agency. I saw an attractive stone house in the midst of a beautiful garden. The trees were covered with an abundance of ripe fruit. The Himalayas in all their majestic glory formed a protective wall beyond the garden. For the first time I was really able to appreciate the beauty of my surroundings and took a deep breath to inhale the clear air. Heavenly! I thought. And this is just the beginning. Hunza lay ahead of me, sixty-eight miles away. My thoughts sailed over the mountains. In a few days I would be in Hunza.

While in Gilgit we were invited to a party given by Mr. Rehman Khan in a lovely garden beneath shady branches of a huge and ancient tree.

About thirty men were seated on both sides of a long table which was bedecked with an array of colorful cookies and cakes. Mr. Rehman Kahn seated me at his right on the bench at the head of the table, introducing me to the handsomely dressed men. I was surprised to find that most of them were named either Ali or Khan, so that if I didn't remember someone's name, I stood a fifty-fifty chance of guessing right.

These men were the dignitaries of Gilgit, doctors from the hospital, teachers from the schools, officers from the army post, subordinates from the office of the political agent. Even though they lived in one of the most isolated corners of the world, they were extremely well read and were able to discuss not only their local problems but affairs of the world as well. Pat Nobbs and I were the only women present. Moslem women seldom participate in such social gatherings. Especially in that remote spot, the women still practice the old customs of the Moslem religion. (However, in the larger cities the women are beginning more and more to follow our Western ways and covering of the face is slowly disappearing in Pakistan. Only a few are still keeping the status of *purdu*, remaining in complete seclusion.) The gathering was a fascinating confrontation of East and West, equally enjoyed by both.

Mr. Rehman Khan, as the political agent in Gilgit, is the sole power in this area of Pakistan. His decisions bear weight of law—even in matters of life and death. I found him holding a court session in his garden the next morning, hearing the case of a man accused of murdering his wife's lover. After the handcuffed man was taken away, Mr. Khan explained the laws governing such cases. The guilt or innocence of one so accused is determined by the distance from which the shot was fired. If the shot is fired from close enough to the scene of the act to give the husband a clear view, then the law exonerates the killer. If, however, the shot is fired at some distance where the husband could not have seen the act clearly, the law declares him to be a murderer. In this case he was declared a murderer and the punishment was death. In some cases it is life imprisonment.

That evening we were dinner guests at Mr. Khan's home. This time I left my fears behind me and thoroughly enjoyed the many delightful dishes set before us, secure that all the vegetables and fruits had come from his beautiful garden and had been painstakingly prepared by his most excellent chef.

Mr. Khan also arranged for a telephone call to His Highness Mir Mohammed Jamal Khan, the ruler of Hunza. This was the first time I had actually made personal contact with the Mir. His voice was friendly and warm, expressing concern about the progress of our group. "All is well," I assured him. "We shall be in Baltit tomorrow!"

"Yes, my sister, my people will help you on the road!"

The next morning, four jeeps and four drivers appeared in the driveway.

Zygmunt was the first to see them. He came out of the house and stood leaning heavily on the porch railing, eyeing the ancient vehicles with incredulity. One of the drivers, a wide-eyed boy of not more than fifteen, flashed an eager smile as the rest of our party came onto the porch to stand beside Zyg.

"Good morning," said the boy in his native tongue, and Mr. Agha, a motion-picture director from the Department of Film of the Government of Pakistan who had joined us in Gilgit, translated.

"Good morning," said Zyg, appraising the other three equally boyish-looking drivers who sat in the decrepit jeeps. He turned his head and looked questioningly at Mr. Agha. "These *children* aren't going to drive us to Hunza?"

Mr. Agha smiled. "I am certain they know how."

Zyg thought about this momentarily and nodded somewhat hesitantly. His eyes were still busy taking note of the jeeps. They did not seem safe enough to ride on the Hollywood Freeway, let alone up the twisting, treacherous sky-high road to Hunza.

Mr. Agha seemed to read his thoughts.

"These were the only jeeps available, Mr. Sulistrowski. As it was, we had great difficulty in obtaining them. If it were not for the influence of the political agent, I am afraid you and your party would have had to either walk or go by pogo stick."

Zyg smiled slightly, very slightly.

We had scarcely reconciled ourselves to the fact that we would be attempting the last and most dangerous phase of our journey with worn-out jeeps and boy drivers, when four other boys appeared from out of the shade of the apricot orchard.

I turned to Mr. Agha. "*Who* are *they?*"

"The drivers' assistants."

"Assistants?"

"Oh, yes. They go with the drivers wherever they go."

"Why?"

"It is absolutely necessary for them to accompany the jeeps."

"What for?" pressed Zyg.

"Because the road to Hunza is unlike any in the world, Mr. Sulistrowski. There are places where the assistants must jump off the jeeps and place rocks under the wheels."

"Nonsense," said Zyg. "I will help the drivers if they need help. We will all help. There are four able-bodied men here . . . five, including you."

"And, if you were to be absolutely safe, you would need twenty more at least. You must understand, there are situations which can arise in the high passes, situations in which you will need every available hand and then wish you had thirty more to help you."

As Zyg exchanged a distraught look with the other members of our group, four other boys appeared. Like the other eight, they were young, friendly and smiling.

"And who are they?" I asked Mr. Agha meekly.

"These are additional assistants sent by the Mir of Hunza."

I am certain that he would have said more, but before he had completed the last sentence four more Hunzakut boys sprouted out of the spreading shade of the apricot orchard. One of the older boys, about nineteen, stepped forward. He was a handsome youth, attired in the native costume of Hunza—baggy-kneed trousers, white homespun shirt fashioned after our Western style, worn outside, and a traditional white woolen cap, with a wide round rim, worn off the face.

"Good morning," he said in English. "The Mir of Hunza has sent us to escort you to our capital, Baltit."

Zyg glowered at Mr. Agha. "And are these the assistants' assistants?"

The Hunzakuts all nodded happily.

"All right, Mr. Agha, now you tell me how we are going to cram four drivers, four drivers' assistants, eight assistants' assistants, seven of us, and thirty-five pieces of luggage into four jeeps. If you can accomplish this feat, then you have my blessings. I will give you no further argument."

With this he turned and went back into the guesthouse.

It was very quiet for a few moments. As we surveyed the army of natives who stood smiling eagerly up at us, Zyg appeared again. He seemed resigned as he said to Mr. Agha, "Do we really need all these men?"

"We do!"

"Then I guess we'll have to take them."

And with that, the four drivers, the four drivers' assistants, the eight assistants' assistants, and the seven members of the expedition began to load the thirty-five pieces of luggage into the four jeeps.

And so, loaded with people and equipment, one by one the jeeps rolled away from the guest house, across the bridge and out onto the road which wound upward into the unknown. What a sight we must have been in that otherwise quiet village of Gilgit. We Americans always create such confusion!

2.

The Road
to Hunza

Within an hour we were in the lower folds of the mountains, climbing steadily upward.

The road became narrower and more primitive as we continued. Occasionally, the sudden turns were so abrupt that the jeeps had to be maneuvered back and forth several times before getting around them. In some places the edge of the road had crumbled away leaving gaping holes, as if some monster had bitten deep into the ledge. Hundreds of feet below we could see the frothy ribbon of the river, and as rocks fell away from the road we watched in awe as they plummeted silently into the depths. Gaps in the road were quickly repaired by our men. Rocks were gathered and the holes filled. Then loose dirt was pounded into the spaces between the rocks to provide a surface that would support the weight of the jeeps.

Among the group from Hunza were several men who had joined us on the road from Gilgit, and we were told that they were over one hundred years old. All of us watched them incredulously as they lightly bounded back and forth carrying heavy boulders. No special consideration was given them by the younger men as they worked side-by-side with men fifty years their junior without faltering or stopping to rest.

Our young drivers appeared to know the road by heart. They warned us in advance of rough sections, of dips, of sudden turns, and they drove their jeeps with a skill that was as impressive as the skill of the pilots who had flown our DC 3 through the great gorges between Rawalpindi and Gilgit. The assistant drivers were called on constantly to aid the progress of the jeeps up the road, which was, in places, just about as wide as our jeep. They would run ahead to guide the drivers around the turns or over the narrower sections of road. It was not unusual for me to look over the side of the jeep and see no road at all, only the dizzying vista of cliff faces which fell away several thousand feet to the river below.

As we drove along, the Hunza men perched atop the luggage chatted helpfully.

"Right here we lost a jeep last year," one boy recalled, then added sadly, "no one was saved."

And another said, "Recently the Mir of Hunza lost a load of very valuable personal belongings somewhere along this stretch. Nothing could be recovered."

Someone remarked, philosophically and only half-joking, "Do not fear. The road gets worse ahead."

And so it did!

As we climbed higher the view became more spectacular. The narrow road seemed to cling to the sheer wall of the mountain. Spreading off to the side was the most magnificent expanse of space I had ever seen in my life. The jagged contours of the peaks rose in a majestic upward thrust of raw stone, capped in white mantles that frayed off into lace against the reddish brown of the mountain shoulders. The sky above seemed like a giant vacuum that was slowly and gradually pulling us up into its clear, vast, blue emptiness. No clouds were visible. It was as if the towering white tips of the ranges had cleared away the distraction of any cloud formation so that their glittering whiteness could stand alone in contrast against the deep blue arch of the sky.

Suddenly a whisper in the distance increased into a muffled, crashing sound. The driver of the lead jeep stopped abruptly and the other drivers did the same. He motioned to the narrow space between the jeeps and the face of the mountain.

"Back! Get back against the mountain!"

Scrambling over luggage, steering wheels, pedals and each other's arms and legs, we managed to flatten ourselves against the cliff. And not a moment too soon!

A few feet in front of our lead jeep, an avalanche of earth and boulders gushed into view, filled the ledge of the road and continued falling into the depths below. Dust filled the air and all sizes of stray rock bounded and rebounded in front of us.

A boulder landed with a roar in the front seat of the jeep where I had been sitting only seconds earlier.

The sound of the falling mass trailed off into the canyon below, leaving us with settling dust and a profound silence. No one spoke. We just looked at each other without saying a word. Zyg was the first to break the silence.

"I want to get pictures of this!"

He climbed back for his camera and went to join the men ahead, who were already beginning to remove the debris from the road. Nobby, Pat and I sat on the edge of the jeeps and began to breathe again. We could hear the sound of feet shuffling along through the ochre dust, could hear the sound of rocks being moved. For a few moments we remained still, savoring the taste of dust in our mouths, savering the bite of the wind against our cheeks, savoring the slightest feeling which told us that we were alive.

I listened to the almost-mocking cry of the Himalayan wind. I do not believe that there is a lonelier sound anywhere in the world. It wailed and moaned like some hopelessly lost creature who will never find a home. And in its wrath it had whipped at the mountainsides, dislodging rocks which, once they had started downward, knocked other rocks loose. Soon thousands of tons of stones were whipping an unchecked pathway into the canyons hundreds of feet below.

"It will take at least six hours to clear the road!" one of the men, who appeared to be in charge of the group, informed us. "We will send a runner to the village we passed a few miles back and see about some food and water for you."

We merely nodded in agreement. The men continued to work on the road. Silently, and with an even, steady pace they cleared away the rocks and patched up the road where sections had been torn away by the slide. The huge stones were handled with an amazing grace. These men from Hunza performed the most arduous task with amazing ease. Nobby, who had some knowledge of civil engineering, said, "It looks like they will have the road ready in six hours at the pace they are going. It's amazing. With our own men and methods it would take days."

Presently we saw one of our drivers coming back up the road. With him was a boy of about twelve years. I can imagine how rapidly word had spread through the village that we had been stranded on the road. How quickly they had come to our aid! Both of them were carrying bundles, which the boy opened and neatly spread out on top of one of the jeeps. There were hard-boiled eggs, chapattis, fresh apricots and goat's milk. When I offered to pay him for the food, he backed away, shaking his head, saying something in Burushaski, the native language of Hunza, which was translated into English for my benefit: "No! Food is given by God to share —not to sell!"

I was filled with compassion for these friendly, unselfish people.

Our appetites were in good form and we proceeded to enjoy the simple, nourishing repast. The chapatti—a flat, round form of bread that looks like the Mexican tortilla—was excellent, and the sweet, sun-ripened apricots the most delicious I had ever tasted.

Of course, there are many instances of strangers being helped in a foreign land by the natives, but here in this section of Pakistan there is so little food that sharing is a true sacrifice.

As the men had predicted, the road was repaired within six hours, but since darkness was beginning to close in we decided to spend the night in the village. There is a guesthouse in every village in Hunza, built by the grandfather of the present Mir for just such emergencies, and the rooms are kept ready for occupancy. This one was a small bungalow in the midst of several apricot trees with a veranda overlooking the mountains.

The only phone in the village was in the home of the local representative of the government, and the interpreter put a call through for me to the Mir of Hunza.

"My beloved sister, I am so glad you are almost here. We are praying for your safety on the journey!"

"Please keep praying," I replied, "I think your prayers were the only thing that saved us this afternoon."

"That was a bad avalanche. I know it has delayed you, but now that the road has been repaired you should be here in time for tea tomorrow afternoon."

"But, Your Highness," I said, surprised at his knowledge of our near catastrophe, "how do you know about the avalanche?"

"We have been watching your progress all day as you were coming up the road. Do you need any additional help? I can send another jeep to meet you."

Thanking him for his concern, I expressed the hope that tomorrow nothing would prevent us from enjoying tea with him.

The rest of the group doubted my story about his having watched us throughout the day. Hunza was still some fifty miles away and it was difficult to understand how the Mir, sitting in his palace, could know every move we were making. I looked up at the dim, jagged silhouette of the mountains against the star-filled sky. Somewhere up there in those majestic peaks unseen eyes had been watching us all day and would continue to follow us tomorrow. Using runners and primitive signaling devices, the Mir could easily receive reports on our progress. I smiled knowingly, somehow reassured.

There was only one room for our overnight stay, so three of our men volunteered to sleep outdoors. The rest of us shared the small accommodations that contained a bed and two narrow couches. There was no bedding, so we curled up in our clothes, pulling our coats around us to keep warm.

The next morning we were all awakened at five o'clock and hot tea was served. The quarters may have been uncomfortable, but the gracious hospitality of our village hosts more than compensated for any inconvenience. Outside, the air was crisp, invigorating and crystal clear, presenting the magnificence of the mountains in the morning sunlight. The colors were intense.

The beginning of that brilliant day seemed almost unreal, and I remember it now with a nostalgic urge to return and sit for hours at the base of those glorious mountains.

It was evident that even the drivers and their helpers felt the beauty of that morning as we pulled away from the village and headed up the road.

The journey was uneventful until we neared the 16,000-foot elevation before the last long descent into the valley of Hunza. We were going up and up. On one side was a wall more than 4000 feet high—on the other a 3000-foot precipice dropping down to the river. The road was becoming even narrower. There was scarcely room for the four wheels to stay on solid ground. One miscalculation would send the jeeps over the edge.

Now the assistant drivers were ahead, kneeling on the ground and guiding the wheels of the jeeps past this treacherous section of the road. The danger of falling was such that everyone was walking, except for the drivers who were inching along the narrow ledge. One man was nearly lost when he slipped and started sliding over. Fortunately a nearby helper grabbed him in time. The rescued man brushed the dust off his trousers and returned immediately to his job of placing rocks under the rear wheels of one of the jeeps to help supply traction for the steep, uphill climb. Not a word was said—just a nod and a smile of thanks to the man who had grabbed him.

When the summit of the pass was reached the men cheered and shook hands with each other. Not once during those two days of unending work had I heard one complaint from these men. Their task had been done quietly and efficiently, working with one another in a tacit understanding of the responsibility of each. The dangers had been accepted as part of the job.

The descent was as steep as our climb had been, and in several places I could not see beyond the front of our jeep. Yet the road itself was better, not quite as narrow, and the surface was smoother. It was still a primitive trail along the edge of the canyon, but by comparison to the rigors of the road up, it seemed like a highway.

I sat back and relaxed after a fashion, but my relief was short-lived. We rounded a turn and discovered that the road had suddenly come to an end.

The Hunza River, which had been at our side for the last two days, spuming and roaring in the bottom of the canyon, now lay ahead. On either side stood two huge brick superstructures similar to the ones on either side of the Golden Gate in San Francisco. But the suspension bridge they had supported was not there. Only a few frayed strands of heavy rope dangled in the wind.

Our driver explained that some years ago, during a tremendous winter storm, the bridge had been blown down, and it probably would be years before it was rebuilt.

"But how do we get across?" I asked.

"The platform will take us," he said, pointing across the river to a rough-planked, raftlike affair suspended by ropes and pulleys from the two heavy cables still intact overhead between the two brick towers.

"I don't believe it!" I gasped.

"Nothing to worry about," replied our driver. "See, they are coming to get us now."

And they were!

"The men on this side pull it over . . . we load . . . then men over there pull it back. It's simple."

"Yes," I said weakly, "very simple!"

The ropes would not have supported the weight of the loaded jeeps so they had to be emptied, the jeeps and the luggage going across in separate trips. For hours the men worked to get the expedition across on this primitive shuttle ferry. Each time the group of men on the opposite side started pulling the platform, it would drop with a sickening lurch to the limit of the stretch in the ropes. Each time I felt that the ropes would not hold and that platform, jeep and men would fall into the rushing torrent of the river below. But it held!

When it came our turn to go across, I was trembling from the anticipation of the ride. I got to the middle of the platform and slipped my fingers through the spaces between the rough planks. I tightened my grip and swore I would not let go until we were on the other side of the river. Then the pull started and the platform seemed to drop away from under me. Someone yelled, "If we go down, try to grab a rock."

We bounced and swayed in the wind above the river. Each time the men pulled the rope the platform jerked and swayed, once tilting so far to one side that I know I would have fallen into the river if I had released my grip on the plank. Up and down, bouncing and swaying, we were slowly—oh, so slowly—pulled across. Not until the edge of the platform was securely tied to the base of the brick towers did I loosen my grip. Then, in three long leaps, I made it to solid ground. Still trembling, I looked at my aching fingers. They were stiff and twisted like claws.

3.

Shangri-La
at Last

Soon the difficulties of the trail were ended. Below was our destination—Baltit, the capital of Hunza.

The long, thin valley stretched from one mountain peak to another, curving about the base of the majestic masses of stone as if the glorious growth of nature had run through the valley in a river of lush vegetation. Yellows, greens and browns were caught in the geometric patterns of the terraces that the natives had built up the sides of the mountains. Brilliant little streams caught the light of the sun and reflected it gaily as they quivered down and across the steps of warm color. The darker green foliage of fruit trees formed verdant borders of lace around some of the fields. Above the valley, above the maze of winding, dusty streets and flat stone houses, above the seemingly endless steps of the terraces, lifting its ice-sheathed summit some 25,500 feet against the blue of the late-afternoon sky, Mount Rakaposhi rose like a gleaming white beacon of welcome.

As our jeeps moved down the road toward the valley, the natives of Hunza could be seen gathering in little groups to watch us pass. They waved and shouted, greeting us with ease, as though they were accustomed to welcoming strangers.

At the outskirts of Baltit we were met by the Crown Prince

Ghazanfar Ali Khan, a tall and handsome young man. Black velvet eyes blended perfectly with his shining black hair. He had a face strong in design and sure in character, with an adult sense of responsibility behind his child-man look, at the age of sixteen. He was accompanied by Prince Ayash Khan, the Mir's brother, a noble gentleman with a broad smile and a gentle voice.

An elegant jeep, spotlessly clean, was very appealing. Without hesitation I took a seat next to the driver—and for the first time in two days stretched my stiff body.

At the gates of the royal grounds waited the younger prince, Amen Khan. Humble and shy, but unusually well poised for his eleven years, he greeted us with the customary *Salaam*, which is followed by a movement of the right hand to the right corner of the forehead.

Some of the natives who had followed us up the road now surrounded the jeeps. Laughing and talking, they crowded close in and around us, inspecting the luggage and motion-picture equipment. Very few outsiders come to this remote land and visitors always cause a stir. Children brought us baskets of apricots and mulberries, politely curtsying before they backed away. The men shouted greetings in their native Burushaski—a tongue of unknown origin. The women could be seen as they watched from the distance, standing on walls or sitting atop their houses. In this Moslem land, women do not publicly mix with men.

"*Salaam!*" was the cry of the Hunzakuts as we followed the royal procession through the unguarded gates of the palace into the garden. Before we had gone much farther, we paused and looked back to where people were still merrily milling about the jeeps.

"Shouldn't we see about posting a guard to watch our equipment?" someone asked.

Mr. Agha smiled, "Remember, you are in Hunza now. There are no thieves here."

A figure was moving toward us through the gardens. He was of average height, with a compact physique clothed in a short-sleeved white shirt worn over dark slacks. As he came closer we could see his full, sun-tanned features. The man extended his hand and shook mine in friendly greeting.

"Welcome to Hunza," he said. "I am Jamal Khan." And then he added, "Welcome home, my sister."

There was no mistaking the man before me.

His Highness the Mir Jamal Khan, the ruler of Hunza, led the way to the palace—a large two-story structure of modern architecture, built of hand-hewn Hunza granite. As we stood in the reception room waiting for the Rani (Queen) Shama-Un-Nahar to make her appearance, I gazed at the artistic arrangement of the lovely furnishings. There was a strange exotic fragrance coming from the large open windows which overlooked the magnificently landscaped gardens. And in the distance one could see the greater part of the valley suddenly ending at the majestic mountain walls.

Then she entered the room—a graceful, beautiful woman with delicate features. She wore a colorful native costume—white silk pajamalike slacks with very wide cuffs at the bottom, and a printed sheath dress cut above the knees, split on both sides like a Chinese coat, with long sleeves. One could see that she adored color. A white chiffon scarf was draped around her. Her skin was light-toned, her brown hair had a touch of red, her eyes were astonishingly dark. When she spoke her voice was as tranquil as her entourage.

"Welcome," she said. "Welcome home."

Then the Rani took us on a tour of what would indeed be our home for the next few months.

Every room in the palace is adorned with priceless collections and gifts from various countries, all tastefully arranged. Persian rugs of unimaginable beauty and value are thrown over the highly waxed floors. The spacious living room leads to a broad, glass-walled terrace which affords a view of the valley below and the towering mountains above.

We were then shown to our rooms. I was invited to stay at the palace, while the rest of our party occupied the guest cottages located in the royal gardens. All of them were furnished comfortably and with dignity. Persian rugs were everywhere and the view of the valley with its terraced fields clinging to the mountain sides, seemed to be part of every vista.

Later, surrounded by the members of the royal family, we were served herb tea and fruit juices. Delicious food was displayed on silver trays. I ate eagerly, downing the hot, invigorating herb tea with relish and drinking several glasses of the fresh fruit juices.

The Mir was amused at my unquenchable appetite and, balancing the cup on his knee, leaned forward and said, "May I suggest, sister, that you keep dinner in mind? We have an excellent cook and the Rani has planned a very special menu for the evening. I know you will be pleased."

I laughed, grateful for the reminder.

Then my eyes rested on the six princesses—Duri Shahwar, Nilofar, Malika, Hussn, Mehr Ul Jamal, Fauzia and Azra—sitting in a semicircle, facing their parents. All were beautiful, closely resembling their mother yet beauties in their own right. Dressed in the same fashion as the Rani, and slender, they moved with an easy grace and showed a limitless vitality.

After bathing, resting and changing I felt like a new person in my sari (which I prefer to any other dress because of its light weight).

We gathered on the glassed-in terrace. Soon a sparkling Hunza-made wine from Hunza-grown grapes was served with nuts, dried apricots and peanuts. At exactly nine o'clock the gong rang for dinner. The long dining table was set with silver and fine rare china. Spaced along its length were silver candelabra supporting a glistening array of pure white candles. Baskets of fruits had been exquisitely arranged by loving hands. The royal insignia of the Mir was embroidered in gold on each piece of linen. The sparkling silver, the shimmering light of the candles, the deep, rich colors of the plump fruit and the mirrorlike surface of the hand-painted china gave a festive, elegant air to the room. It was like dining at the most elegant restaurant in Beverly Hills, not at all like taking a meal in a secluded Asian valley on the roof of the world.

Dinner was delicious. The food was artfully served and consisted of a mint soup, a tender, delicately spiced lamb curry with rice and fresh vegetables, a green salad prepared plain with a side dressing of grape vinegar and apricot-kernel oil, so that each person could suit his own taste. For dessert there was ice cream made from snow brought down from the nearby Himalayan glaciers and sweetened with dried, puréed apricots. And, of course, a variety of chapattis, the famous Hunza bread.

After dinner we gathered in the drawing room and relaxed with the easy comfort that always follows a delicious meal enhanced by the congeniality of a friendly group. The Mir discussed politics at length and proved to be extremely well informed on world affairs. He listens daily to shortwave newscasts from all over the world and subscribes to many leading magazines and newspapers of various countries.

At ten o'clock everyone usually retires. The electricity, supplied by a small diesel generator (for palace use only), goes off at ten-thirty. Lack of fuel does not permit this luxury of light to last more than three hours each evening.

Alone in my room, I opened the window beside my bed and looked out into the vastness of the night. The moon was full and the stars were brilliant in the clear darkness of the sky. A deep silence lay upon the valley. Over all was a pervading sense of harmony and tranquility, combined with the intangible mysteries of this high-mountain fairyland.

At seven o'clock the next morning a neatly dressed butler brought my breakfast on a tray. For at least an hour I sipped at the vigorous herb tea, ate tasty bread made from whole-grain wheat and enjoyed delicious apricot jam which, despite its sweetness, contained no sugar. The Hunzakuts have no sugar other than the natural sugar of the land. Their fruits are astonishingly sweet and of magnificent quality. The butter for my bread had been made from goat's milk.

My double-sized bed stood along a large window facing Mount Rakaposhi. Persian rugs were spread on the shining waxed floor. Two easy chairs upholstered in red velvet added comfort and elegance. The room was in the left wing of the palace, on the same floor as the living quarters of the Mir and Rani.

I was entranced with my new home. There were two other windows on the opposite wall, letting the sun in, which gaily played on the many objects inside the room. My private bathroom had modern plumbing facilities and cold running water. Hot water steamed in waiting buckets. I washed and dressed.

At my window I drew hungry draughts of the crisp, clean air, smelled the brisk aroma of racing rivers and gazed at the high, impregnable mountaintops.

In the small village below I could see the natives beginning their day's work, moving through the waist-high wheat. The colors of the land were brilliant in the intense rays of the morning sun. The ribbon of the valley bottom stretched out below me, the terraced fields rising on either side.

Yet I knew that Hunza had not always been the peaceful valley that it was on that day.

LORE AND LEGEND OF HUNZALAND

The Hunzakuts tell a legend about the first settlers to come to their valley many centuries ago. Three soldiers who deserted the army of Alexander the Great escaped to the valley, bringing their Persian wives with them. The small group prospered in the ideal conditions of this earthly paradise, and within several generations a thriving community had been established. Warlike in nature, they fought off all invaders who attempted to trespass upon the land they had claimed as their own. These early Hunzakuts are said to have repelled not only the great Genghis Khan, but later, the armies of the English as well. The towering peaks of the Himalayan mountains surrounding the valley provided a natural fortress.

In their early days, the Hunzakuts were feared along the trade routes through the neighboring ranges. For centuries the main route between Sinkiang and Kashmir was the scene of their marauding. Chinese traders agreed to pay tribute to Hunza so that their caravans—laden with silks, tea and porcelain—might go unmolested over the passes to India, then return to Cathay with spices, jewels, ivory and gold.

The primitive Hunzakuts were very agreeable when it came to accepting tribute, but were not so quick to keep their word. As soon as the Chinese pack trains would enter their territory, they would scale the surrounding peaks and hurl huge boulders down upon the road, sending the helpless caravans into the dizzying chasms hundreds of feet below. Then, at their leisure, the Hunzakuts, like gleeful pirates, would recover their booty.

Not until Nazim Khan, the grandfather of the present Mir, came to rule did the terroristic raids finally cease. The Mir has told me, "At the age of twelve a brilliant child and the favorite son, Nazim convinced his father that fighting and killing and stealing could not possibly be the basic principle of life. On the contrary, God created men to live in peace and harmony with each other, and the time should come for our people to abide the law and the wish of God. He was a very unusual child . . . rather a little man at his age.

"His father, my great-grandfather, confessed to him that he would like to make peace with the neighbors; however, no one would believe him anymore. Too many promises had been made by our ancestors and they were never kept. Nevertheless, Nazim Khan wouldn't give up and continued to plead with his father to try again.

"Finally a dispatch was sent to Gilgit (at that time part of India and part of the British Empire) with the message that the Mir of Hunza was ready to sign a peace treaty. The note was accepted by the English officials under one condition, that the young son would be sent to Gilgit and kept as a hostage until the exchange of documents took place.

"Nazim begged his father to accept this and went to Gilgit. The treaty was signed, and after ten days the boy returned safely to Hunza. The promise of peace has never been broken.

"Soon after that incident, Nazim Khan became Mir, and for over one hundred years peace has reigned in the land. The brigand glory of those early days is now only a memory and a heritage of stories that are told to the children by the older men with a faraway look in their eyes."

The Hunzakuts are different from the other races living in this part of the world. Their features are Caucasian and they rather resemble southern Europeans. Their language, Burushaski, is not related to any spoken tongue and its origin is still a mystery to scholars. It is highly complicated, having sixteen plural forms, and its words resemble no other words I have ever heard.

GARDENS OUT OF STONE

Centuries ago, the men of Hunza had to devise a way to create more arable land. It stood to reason that crops could not grow out of the solid rock of mountains. But there was no reason why soil could not be brought and placed upon the rocky areas. On the slopes which were chosen for cultivation, the men dug a horizontal ditch, then placed rocks around them. Soil was laid over the freshly hewn foundation—earth which had to be carried one basketful at a time from the silt-rich river-bottom land some 2000 feet or more below the terrace. A retaining wall from 4 to 8 feet high was built around the terrace so the soil would not be washed away and the water would not seep out.

Irrigation channels were coursed so that melting snowwater constantly seeping down from the glaciers could be caught and held. The excess water is trapped in a deep, rockbound gorge.

The Hunzakuts built this vast and successful terrace system completely without the aid of any tools, save their own primitive implements.

Now, thousands of years later, the men of Hunza still use this system of terracing. When new land is needed, another step in the mountain is constructed.

Apparently this method of agriculture is the oldest form of land cultivation in the world. It is known that in the towering realm of the Andes, long before the Incas ruled Peru, a race of people lived who perfected exactly the same agricultural system as is used by the Hunzakuts.

In 1916, O. F. Cook of the Bureau of Plant Industry of the United States Department of Agriculture wrote an article in the *National Geographic* magazine entitled "Staircase Farms of the Ancients," from which I quote: "Agriculture is not a lost art, but must be reckoned as one of those which reached a remarkable development in the remote past and afterward declined. The system of the ancient Peruvians enabled them to support large populations in places where modern farmers would be helpless."

The terraces give one an overwhelming impression of grandeur. They are fields literally hewn out of a mountainside, fields which our Western engineers would have deemed impossible to construct. Yet there they are, not only prospering but yielding some of the most nutritious produce in the world. The Hunzakuts are proud of their fields, and they are proud and happy to work them.

It is strange to realize that two completely alien civilizations, one now extinct, could without ever knowing of each other's existence construct practically identical agricultural systems. The Peruvian society which constructed terraces has left no records. Their existence might never have been noted if it had not been for their magnificent terraces, which are still in use today. The walls of these ancient terraces were made to fit so perfectly that a woman would find it impossible to slip even a hairpin through a chink between the stones.

Although the megalithic people to whom the Peruvian terraces are attributed have been lost to recorded history, their genius of construction and their magnificent, passionate love for the perfection of the art of stonework remains with us today as an epitaph.

The Hunzakuts, like the vanished megaliths, have reached perfection in the art of building with stone. Without the aid of even so simple a modern tool as a hammer, they have built homes and mosques and irrigation canals and terraces which will, I am sure, be standing when the last blizzard darkens the Himalayas and earth-men have fled a dying planet to take up residence in other galaxies.

4.

The Land of
Just Enough

The Mir was smiling at me, indulgently.

"But if you haven't any guards," I persisted, "aren't you leaving yourself vulnerable to attack?"

"There are no guards stationed at my palace for the same reason that there are no jails or banks in Hunza. What good are banks in a land that has no money? What use are jails in a land without crime? And what service can guards do a man who has no enemies?"

"No enemies at all?"

"Only the elements of nature, but we have learned to combat them."

"And no money?"

"There are no banks in Hunza. Money as such is of no importance. There are no taxes, fees, licenses or duties, so my people don't have much use for money. We have no stores to shop in and the land cannot be bought or sold. It is inherited and must remain in the family. (Usually the son who loves agriculture most gets possession of the land.) If there are other sons in the family, then they may turn to various occupations—becoming mountain porters, trail runners or guides. Also, recently many of our young men began to join the Gilgit Scouts of the Pakistani army and protect the borders along the mountain region. Some of them become tailors, goldsmiths, weavers or help farmers with various jobs. As a rule no one owns more than five acres of land, enough for one family to take care of."

"And what about you, Your Highness?" I asked.

"I own over 300 acres," he told me. "However, I am slowly giving it away, parcel by parcel, to some young men who haven't inherited any land. No one needs money. If something happens to a villager, all the neighbors stand by to offer a helping hand. If a man loses a horse, a neighbor will loan him a horse. A silver Pakistani rupee is worth twenty cents, and a Hunzakut prefers this coin to five- or ten-rupee paper notes. Silver can be safely put away. Also, a large paper note would be hard to change. I take care of all the import and export of absolutely necessary goods such as tools, cattle and horses, and other things made out of steel and so forth. Most of these transactions are done by exchange. Caravans coming through Hunza from China carrying goods to Pakistan or India leave cotton cloth, kitchen utensils, silk and other things for fruit, grains, lodging and food if the traders spend a night in the valley. There is no money and no poverty. Education is free to all. Food is often scarce, but no one starves. We have the greatest gift of all . . . our health. The diseases of modern civilization are unknown here, including cancer."

The conversation was interrupted by the telephone. Every evening the *arbab* (head of a village) reports to the Mir and tells him of the day's happenings. There is one phone in every village for this purpose only. The calls are always made at about the same time, so as we watched the Mir we knew that he was holding a multiway conversation.

After he hung up, he smiled and told us that his people wished us well.

"Tell me," one of our group asked him, "don't you people ever get lonely up here?"

"We are the happiest people in the world," the Mir answered without hesitation. "We have just enough of everything but not enough to make anyone else want to take it away. You might call this 'the happy land of just enough.'"

The Rani, sitting opposite the Mir at a bench near the grand piano (which twenty men had carried up the treacherous Himalayan pass as a gift to the Mir's grandfather), smiled shyly in approval.

For years she had lived in *purdu*, but lately the Mir had allowed his beloved Queen and the other women of Hunza to uncover their faces after the modern fashion.

Although she has accompanied her husband on many trips to the far corners of the world, the Rani has remained almost painfully shy. Nevertheless, she is like an ineluctable magnet—a quiet, undeniable central fire. And her children, her husband, her servants and her friends have all succumbed to her quiet charm.

The Rani has set a pattern of existence which the Hunza women follow as anxiously as American women follow the styles of fashion set by film stars. However, just as the Rani is the true Queen of her state and household, so, too, each Hunzakut woman is the queen of her own domain.

During our stay in Hunza the Rani was always dressed exquisitely, choosing pastel blues, violet, reds and occasionally black. One day she wore white silk ballooning pantaloons under a knee-length blue lace sheath dress, and a pillbox hat daintily embroidered in many colors with a long white chiffon scarf draped across it.

A wonderful hostess, the Rani was full of surprises. Usually we women gathered at five o'clock every afternoon to take tea with her. One afternoon she brought out a record player and surprised us with the latest American records. Her daughters danced to this music and improvised lovely choreography in Hunza style.

Respected and loved throughout the valley, the Rani is of great help to her husband.

"At least once a year," said the Mir, "the Rani and my family accompany me on a tour of inspection throughout the state. While I counsel with the elders and see my people, the Rani visits with the women and listens to their needs. We camp outdoors in many places and it is lots of fun. Even our English governess, Mrs. Hansen, who is in her seventies, joins us on some of these trips. Before she came to live with us, she was told in London that she had a bad heart and should give up working and lead a peaceful life. Being a nurse by profession and a very active person, it wasn't easy for her to do. She returned to Pakistan, where she was born and had lived for many years. After I heard her story, I offered to have her come to Hunza and stay with us.'·

"But, Your Highness, with a bad heart, and over these mountain passes?"

He smiled. "Yes, she withstood the dangerous trip over the mountain passes from Gilgit and has made it twice since then. Originally her condition was such that she was not expected to live more than a few months. She has been with us now for two years. Since she came to Hunza, her health has improved. Whether it is our food, our excellent water or the pure air, I cannot say what has help her. It must be a combination of everything."

Besides English and Burushaski, the Mir speaks Persian, Urdu, Arabic and the dialects of half a dozen neighboring princely states fluently. He was educated in a British school in neighboring Gilgit.

The Mir's large library contains a collection of fine books, and runners bring mail and news up from Gilgit every other day. He also subscribes to many national magazines and is well informed in world politics. His mornings are reserved for business and meetings with his elders to discuss affairs of state. The afternoons are set aside for sports and recreation. His Highness knows how to be happy, and so does his family.

His brother Prince Ayash acts as his assistant and counsel. A jovial and friendly person, he is always on hand to assist the Mir. He is very happy in his dedication to matters of state, and his humor kept us constantly entertained.

One day I wandered through the cemetery, located on a knoll not far from the palace. A sparkling white wall that guards the tombs of many former mirs glistened in the early-morning light. It was scarcely five o'clock. I heard a low chanting. Then I saw the Mir. He was praying at the tomb of his grandfather. The Koran, their Bible, was in his hand. He didn't see me, and I quickly retreated so as not to disturb him.

Later the Mir told me that he goes daily to the cemetery to pray, asking his grandfather for guidance and blessings.

"Our people believe that after death an angel joins the person in the grave to review the records of life, and therefore the graves are built large enough for two people—in a sitting position."

As days passed, I learned more and more about these people, and I came to respect and love them. But I couldn't help wondering how long Hunza could remain peaceful, with so much political unrest just outside its borders. I questioned the Mir.

"All I can do is hope," he smiled. "As long as we don't have anything valuable, I don't think anybody will want to bother with us. Our roads are dangerous, we have no hotels, no restaurants, no movies, no television, and no gold or oil. So what can anyone get from us? A few years back I was alarmed by a prospector who thought he had found a rich vein of gold near Baltit. Fortunately he was wrong. Gold would have been the end of Hunza and our way of life."

5.

Growing Up
Happy

"In Hunza there is no juvenile delinquency," said His Highness.

"And that then is why you have no crime and no jails?"

"Precisely that. You see, here in Hunza children are taught to obey from the very start. Discipline is a natural thing and respect for age, property and wisdom is inherent.

"Parents have the greatest opportunity to offer guidance to their children on the path to a healthy maturity of mind as well as body. But it calls for certain sacrifices on the part of the parents. It calls for wisdom, strength, understanding and, above all, patience—also love, real love, all that any human being can give. Only parents can have learned what to do and what not to do.

"There is a job designed for everyone, and these jobs are done with devotion and without resentment. The children have learned to combine work and play. They are never in the way of their parents.

"Here in Hunza I never hear a mother scolding or bribing her children, or threatening them.

"Negative thoughts must be put aside in Hunza, where children play in the shadows of the great peaks and scamper along the cliff-faces like young goats.

"Youngsters are taught respect for the land but not fear of it, for when fear is present, reasoning generally vanishes into the whirlpool of panic. Panic, as we all know, usually has disaster following eagerly in its wake, not only for the youngsters but for the adults as well. Because Hunzakut mothers are only too aware of the latter factors, they are not forced to hover over their offspring to make certain they will not disobey.

"By the time a Hunza baby is old enough to walk and is strong enough to tramp along the mile-high roads, he must be able to watch out for himself. The women are far too busy cooking, working in the fields and traipsing to the river to do their laundry to maintain a constant lookout. It is impossible for them to devote hours just to the care of their children, therefore the children learn the meaning of responsibility at about the same time they learn to crawl.

"In Hunza it is not necessary to apply strategy to get cooperation from children, or for that matter from adults. Cooperation is needed, and so it is given. There is an unspoken conviction in this high-mountain realm where the elements so dominate the way of life—no one can succeed unless everyone succeeds."

For a moment the Mir was silent, looking out the window which was facing Mount Rakaposhi, deep in thought.

After a while he continued, "While the girls stay close to home, learning how to cook and sew and embroider and take care of the younger members of the family, the boys attend school. The Aga Khan, the spiritual leader of the Ismaili sect, [a sect of the Moslem religion] to which my people belong, has had schools built in every village, and for the first time in the entire history of Hunza, the male children are being given an opportunity to learn about the world which lies beyond their valley. They embrace this chance to gain knowledge of the world in which they live, coming to attend classes and participate in various activities ranging from the casual singing of native songs to exercises to serious study."

The boys meet outdoors on the plaza to sing and pray together for an hour under the direction of the teacher. Then they exercise for an hour. Their exercises are quite strenuous and, watching them, one has to admire their conviction that physical fitness is part of their education. Then they return to the schoolhouse to attend classes, which are conducted for two hours. Pencils and paper are not readily available, so the teacher writes words on the blackboard and the students repeat them, learning by heart. They study four languages simultaneously: Urdu (spoken in Pakistan), Persian, English and Burushaski, their native language. The children learn these languages quite easily.

In the afternoon they return home to share their newly acquired knowledge with their families. There is no coeducation in Hunza. However, Karim, the grandson of the late Aga Khan and the present spiritual leader of Hunza, has recently established the first girl's school in Hunza and now even some of the girls are studying.

"The Hunzakut families are extremely close," said the Mir, "yet, to your Western way of thinking, I imagine the relationship between mother and child could be thought of as strange."

"In a way it could," I agreed. I remembered only that afternoon walking through the village with my eight-year-old Hunzakut guide, who was giving me a lesson in the native language of Burushaski. My young guide and I were having a delightful time. He would point at things and say them in Burushaski and then make me repeat after him. Then a woman came toward us on the road. My guide paused long enough in his instruction to lift his small arm to his forehead and greet her with a casual *salaam*. She smiled and returned his greeting as she continued on her way, never slowing her pace. I would have thought nothing of this brief passing, except that the woman was very lovely.

"What a beautiful woman," I said, more to myself than to my guide. "I wonder who she is?"

"Oh," said my little guide. "That was my mother returning from the fields. We live up that path." He turned and pointed off, and I caught a definite look of unconcealed pride and admiration in his oval, handsome face as he traced the movement of his mother until she disappeared from view.

She had not stopped to embrace her child, nor had she questioned him about where he had been, where he was going or if he would be home for dinner.

She trusted him implicitly. This is not at all unusual. Every Hunza child is well adjusted and happy because he is trusted and knows the meaning of responsibility.

There is no jealousy in the domestic life of Hunzakut husbands and wives. Each women is sure of her husband's respect and love. She lives in perfect peace within her own realm and is able to create happiness for her family and security for her children. Divorce is rare, therefore children are seldom confronted by the awesome and painful problem of having to choose between one parent and the other.

Parents and teachers alike encourage the children to develop initiative, individuality and the qualities of leadership. Hunza children are healthy—emotionally and physically—and healthy children are happy children, especially when they are shown that they have a definite place in society, that they are not misfits, that they are an integral part of everyday existence and that their thoughts and actions are of concern and value not only to themselves but to everyone in their community. In Hunza, children are encouraged to be seen *and* heard. Because of this, they are more than eager to direct their energies into constructive rather than destructive channels.

"Tell me about the parents in your country," the Mir said.

"In my opinion," I answered, "there are four types of Western parents who, even when trying their best, often destroy the lives of their children.

"First we have very young parents who married while still in their teens. These parents, generally between the ages of seventeen and twenty-two, are frightened by the responsibility put before them. A child is indeed a precious gift and they realize this only too well. They doubt their adequacy to handle the situation so they turn to innumerable articles, magazine stories, handbooks and books for information on child training. Naturally, since everyone has his own ideas on 'bringing up baby,' the young couple is thoroughly confused, and so is the baby. By the time the child of such a couple is five years old it is completely undisciplined and as confused by its actions and motives as are its parents.

"Then we have the parents who are too quick to judge their child, to reprimand and to punish. Junior is raised under two pairs of iron thumbs. He is taught never to speak out of turn, never to dirty his clothes and never to venture off on his own. A child raised in such an environment becomes resentful and actually looks for opportunities to disobey.

"And then there are the parents who are afraid to administer discipline for fear of losing their child's love. All this misguided conception achieves is that the child inevitably loses respect for his

parents and develops an overgrown sense of authority and importance. In short, he will probably strut about like 'Little Caesar,'
telling his parents to 'shut up,' 'mind your business,' and the like.

"There is still another type—this is the 'devoted' parent. I once
knew a very fine man who, when his wife died, was left with a
five-year-old boy. The man gave his entire life to bringing up the
child. Although he did not realize it, after all of this self-sacrifice
he came to look upon the boy not as a son but as a piece of property. When at twenty-two the boy took a wife, the father saw in
his daughter-in-law a competitor. He made no attempt to understand or get to know the girl. Instead he openly criticized her background, her education and her physical appearance. He berated his
son, saying that he was ungrateful, and that he had used instead
of loved his father. In truth, although the boy did love his father,
he had actually contemplated marriage as the way to free himself
from his domineering influence. He had married the first woman
who came into his life."

The Mir nodded. "Ah, yes, such extremes can never cause anything but heartbreak in the long run. In Hunza such extremes are
never heard of. There is only one way to raise a child—he is taught
respect for his parents, respect for the society in which he dwells
and respect for himself. Once he has learned these three simple
things he cannot become a delinquent. A Hunza child shares a deep
and unspoken understanding with his parents. They give him wisdom, strength, patience and love. He is never censured, but if he
does wrong he is corrected. From the moment he is born, he is
respected as an individual. There is no mold into which he must
force himself. The only form to which he must adhere are the rules
of his society, a society which is strong because of its will to support the strength and freedom of the individual.

"It is often said that children are but slightly varying reflections
of their parents. This is not true. We must not forget that a child,
although born of his mother's womb, once severed from the um-
bilical cord is an individual entity.

"In Hunza, where nature and her forces so dominate the way of
life, parents know that it is not enough to train their children to
survive and be comfortable. The material wealth which a man
accumulates in his lifetime cannot go with him beyond the grave.
It is necessary that children be taught to find their happiness ac-

cumulating wealth of a different sort—the wealth of mental and spiritual values which are theirs throughout eternity."

In Hunza, when a child raises his eyes to the soaring majesty of Mount Rakaposhi, his face wears a delighted smile. He could not be happier if he had stumbled on the lost treasure of Solomon. Or perhaps he has found this treasure. Surely Solomon the Wise must have found the immeasurable treasure of the little things—of the fragrance which accompanies the dawn, of the sound of the morning birds, of the wind moving through rainwashed trees and of snowclouds wafting silently away from the summits of great mountains. The treasure of life, of sight, of sound, of all the five senses . . . the treasure of the gift of life: in Hunza this is the greatest treasure of all.

6.

The Woman's World

In Hunza I witnessed a scene I shall never forget.

Each year the Mir performs a mass wedding ceremony. One day during the first week in December is chosen for the occasion.

It is difficult for anyone to forget a wedding anniversary in Hunza, since everyone gets married at the same time.

During our stay, however, the Mir planned a wedding, out of season, as a special celebration for two young men who were leaving Hunza to join the Gilgit Scouts—a garrison of the Pakistani army which protects the surrounding Himalayan peaks.

It was the first Hunza wedding ceremony ever filmed. Since the ceremony traditionally takes place in December there had been no previous chance of a stranger being present, for the roads are usually impassable during the winter season.

I persuaded the Mir to ask the women to attend the "out-of-season" festivities. The invitation was extended to them at the very last moment, but they lost no time in dashing to their homes and donning their best clothes. They primped and combed their luxuriant hair, patted apricot oil on their faces, put on every bit of jewelry they could find and draped exquisite shawls over their pillbox hats. Then, with excitement-flushed faces, they lined the rooftops to view the wedding ceremony and the ensuing dance. They, like the beads which they so adore, were like a multicolored magnificent necklace of happiness as they stood against the blue Himalayan sky.

The Queen, the princesses and I were watching from the terraces of the royal summer residence in Altit, where the annual wedding ceremonies takes place, facing the yard, which had been decorated for the occasion. We had a clear view of the inside of the houses through the one wall which remains open to the veranda of each house. The women, unaware that they were being watched, attended to their grooming. It was obvious that each woman was very conscious of her appearance, and although she would be witnessing the festivity from the roof above, she still wanted to be attractive. This demonstration convinced me that no matter where a woman is, she never forgets to be beautiful and feminine.

MARRIAGE, HUNZA STYLE

Marriage is sacred to the Hunzakuts, and since it takes place in wintertime and all the chores have been finished, they have time to really celebrate for a few days, drinking their homemade grape wine, dancing and singing.

The grooms perform a special saber dance. They usually wear ornamental headdresses adorned with jewelry, which is a wedding present for their brides.

They exhibit the aggressive nature of their warlike ancestors during the dance. These attitudes become apparent only during competitive games and ceremonial dancing.

The Mir told me, "The groom's mother spends the honeymoon with the newlyweds, acting as guide and teacher. Marriage is too important to be left to chance."

I smiled, but made no comment.

In the old days the parents had the right to ordain who should marry whom, how, why, when and where. There were no two ways about it. But today, although the marriages are still decided by the parents, the children very definitely have something to say about it. The proposed bride and groom may view each other from a distance and, if they seem not to be at all attracted to one another, a sincere talk with the parents might change the plans. Even the two princesses, the daughters of the Mir, did not actually meet their grooms until their wedding day. At first, I must admit, this custom did not seem exactly fair to me. I asked the Rani how she had gone about selecting husbands for her daughters.

"I tried to choose boys who could make my daughters happy," she said, smiling slightly. "Boys who would fit well into the family surroundings . . . also be good providers."

In Hunza the parents bring the groom to meet the bride on the wedding day. There is no courtship in Hunza, but there is virtually no divorce, either. Evidently the mothers and fathers make good choices.

THE HUNZA WOMAN AS WORKER, WIFE AND MOTHER

The women of Hunza share the responsibility of bringing home the beans, so to speak. They work side-by-side with their men in the fields. In the villages, the men who do not choose to work the fields attend to such important jobs as weaving material, sewing the heavy garments which must be worn during the bitter winter months and milling the flour. In Hunza each individual is allowed to choose his own profession. There is work for all.

The women have no time for idle chitchat. Each day is well planned, and each task must be accomplished. Things are done in a quiet and competent manner. There is no tension or anxiety. The usual drone of our society, "Oh, well, I can always do it to-morrow," is never heard here. The Hunza housewife goes about her duties without being concerned about what the neighbors are doing. Yet, if a friend or neighbor should need help, she is ready and willing to pitch in.

I have seen Hunzakut women over seventy and eighty doing physical chores without showing the slightest signs of fatigue. And the gardener's wife at eighty trudged twice daily up the 1200-foot pathway to her home above the palace.

The women of Hunza are slim, erect and walk with a light glide that makes them seem as though they were walking on delicate puffs of clouds which might very well give way if they should take too heavy a step.

Although the women of Hunza are restricted in their public activities, as all Moslem women are, they are deeply respected by their men. Not only do they perform the household duties of women the world over and work in the fields along with their husbands, but when it comes to recreational activities, although you won't find a Hunzakut woman participating in them, she'll be there, watching from a distance. In the past few years, many of the old traditional restrictions of Moslem law have been dropped— the Hunza women today wear no veils and go about freely. As time goes on, undoubtedly they will assume a more active role in the society of their country.

It is said in Hunza that childbirth is a woman's duty, proves her fortitude, determination and good health. If a woman is in perfect health she will, as a rule, have no difficulties in delivering a child. The women are so healthy that they need no medical assistance at all.

The Rani told me that shortly after the delivery of one of her girls, her father appeared at the palace. He had come all the way from a neighboring district some distance away. Since the Rani was not expecting him, and since no man is allowed to enter a woman's bedroom except her husband, she promptly got out of bed and walked down the stairs to greet her father, saying, "A few minutes ago you became a grandfather again."

After the birth of an infant, the mother breast-feeds a baby boy for three years and a baby girl for two years. During this time, to protect herself from pregnancy, she stays away from her husband and lives without any emotional disturbance. It works very well in Hunza, but I don't recommend it for our way of living. However, certain modifications could be incorporated in our pattern, and the young mother could learn more about her responsibilities while pregnant.

Dr. Robert C. McCarrison, a British surgeon who served in the Gilgit area and spent seven years with the Hunzakuts, wrote: "In Hunza, infants are reared as nature intended them to be . . . at the mother's breast. If this source of nourishment fails, they die; and at least they are spared the future of gastrointestinal disorders which so often have their origin in the first bottle."

It is possible that breast-feeding has a great influence not only on the physique, but also on the mental attitude and development of the child. Yet, even in our Western world, with mothers who do breast-feed their infants, the infant mortality rate is high. In Hunza it is practically nonexistent. Perhaps this is because the Hunza mother has better diet and, consequently, a superior-quality milk.

Hunza children get a magnificent start in life, and this good start is undoubtedly the result of the excellent diet of their mothers. Teeth are another indication of the quality of the nutrition of the mother before the birth of a child, as they form while the foetus is in the womb and are within the gums at birth. Hunza children have perfect white teeth and healthy gums, and they have neither toothpowders, toothpastes nor toothbrushes. They clean their teeth with little twigs which they chew until one end resembles a brush, and with this they clean in and around the teeth and massage the gums. The massage is very important, as it brings blood to the surface and keeps the gums healthy and active.

We are familiar with the widespread defectiveness of teeth in civilized societies. But the Hunza children don't eat sweets, ice cream or drink soft drinks. They eat lots of fresh fruit or chew on dried fruit, as well as on raw carrots and other raw vegetables. And as for beverage, they drink the natural, pure water rich in all the minerals brought down from the glaciers. And they eat sparingly. There is not enough food for them to become gluttons.

BEAUTY IS AS BEAUTY DOES

The old cliché "women are women" holds as firmly in Hunza as it does in New York or London or Timbuktu. Despite the fact that she has been isolated from society for centuries, she has still managed to fully maintain her femininity.

Beauty, as with women the world over, is important to the women of Hunza. They are always neat and always striving to better their appearance.

Jewelry captivates them. Anklets, necklaces, bracelets, earrings . . . they love them all as long as they glitter and sparkle with color. Oh, how they love color!

Every woman and girl wears a pert little pillbox hat perched jauntily atop her head. This hat is embroidered in a profusion of color and vivid design. You might even go so far as to call them "happy hats," because it is virtually impossible to look at one without smiling with delight.

Over the hat is worn a long sweep of chiffon. This is draped about their heads and allowed to flow over their bodices and shoulders. In the days when Moslem women covered their faces, this chiffon served as a quick coverup when a man wandered into sight. Now, however, as this old tradition is slowly being abolished, the women of Hunza retain this graceful, almost Grecian headgear, but are not so quick to hide their faces or to conceal their remarkable complexions, which they attribute to the wonders of apricot oil.

The women and girls seem to personify the mother-and-daughter team. They not only wear the same type of hat, but their entire costume is identical. The dress of the women consists of slacks which look like a cross between pajamas and bellbottom trousers. These slacks are generally made of white cotton, linen or silk. Over them is worn a sheath dress which is highly reminiscent of the Chinese mandarin coat, with deep slits on either side.

The predominant color in Hunza is red, for it is the brightest and most popular. Wherever you go, through the villages or to the fields, or to the ancient stone fortresses high on the mountainsides, it seems as though some playful god has adorned the landscape in this vibrant color.

Like all women, the women of Hunza just can't dress up enough. But in Hunza this complaint is justified, as women generally do not attend any of the festivities or public functions.

In Hunza the women do not concern themselves with the passing of time, for time is not measured by clocks or calendars. Time is judged by the changing of the seasons, and each season brings the feeling of newness, not a fear that time is slipping irrevocably away. In the West on the other hand, where lives are dominated by clocks and calendars, we tend to view each passing moment as a little piece of life which has cruelly slipped away from us, never to return. Each such slipping bit of time brings us closer to old age and, ultimately, to death. We worry so much about growing old that we actually increase the process. We purchase creams and spend countless dollars in the vague hope of erasing unwanted lines. Then, after we have applied these semisolid face-lifters, instead of going about our business and giving them a chance to work we stand in front of the mirror and worry so hard that new wrinkles are born . . . not from age, but from worry. We may not realize it, but we are actually worrying ourselves into early graves.

The women of Hunza have lovely complexions. And their children have beautiful skin—no acne or other disfiguring blemishes. Of course, their food is simple, healthful, and they do not eat sugar, white or raw, or any other of our "civilized delights"—ice cream, candy, soft drinks.

It might be a very comforting thought to learn that our skin ages not because of advancing years but for a completely different reason. Wrinkles and lines which begin to etch themselves into the film-laden outer skin in adulthood are accentuated by the daily deposit of atmospheric dust, dirt, grease and grime to which the facial skin is hourly exposed. Physiology tells us that waste fluid exudes from the ducts of the body, covering the entire skin area. This fluid contains a gum base that remains on the skin after the fluid content of the eliminated waste material has evaporated. These combined deposits adhere to the outer facial skin and become embedded deep within the skin pores. A filmlike coating gradually forms which becomes accumulative as we approach adulthood.

There are two sides to the facial skin, the inner and the outer tissues:

1. Blood feeds the skin from within. The inner skin receives its nourishment from the capillaries, which should have an unrestricted flow of blood to wash out accumulated toxic waste materials.

2. Oxygen feeds the blood from without. Our skin pores are tiny nostrils which serve the purpose of inhalation. They expand to discharge waste materials and to aid in oxygenation.

Heavy creams clog and seal pores until they cease to function normally. When the pores become clogged externally, the intake of oxygen is shut off, which affects the skin's coloring, therefore the skin pores must be emptied of waste materials before they can resume the task which nature assigns them. It may come as a surprise to learn that lines, wrinkles and shadows form in this skin film and not, as is generally believed, in the true skin itself.

There are products on the market which will remove the extra skin-building weight and pressure of the external deposits, and then stimulate the blood's circulation to the skin tissues to help restore them to normal functioning. Many of my friends have experimented with this principle and have experienced spectacular results.

Today many of the cosmetics are prepared from pure foods. Avocados, papayas, almonds, honey, herbs, apricot oils, minerals and vitamins are refined, balanced and blended to restore, enhance and preserve your beauty.

We are indeed fortunate that science has come forth with new and wonderful discoveries and has perfected oils from pure foods which are beneficial to skin care and not harmful to delicate face and neck tissues. Recently I paid a visit to a laboratory engaged in making these natural cosmetics in El Monte, California, and I was amazed to find baskets of lemons, oranges, apricots, avocados and papayas, not to mention a multitude of other types of fruits and vegetables.

To keep that "young" look aglow, you must also avoid wrinkles and a drooping neck, for as we all know these two things are always thought of as a direct key to telling one's age. Actually, this is not true, your neck and face have very few oil glands, therefore, not enough care, also too much exposure to sun or wind, or cold air, can easily cause drying and wrinkling of the upper facial skin. Therefore, you must constantly make sure that these areas are never left without a generous application of these nourishing natural oils.

HEARTH, HOME AND DAILY ROUTINE

The Hunza homes are built of stone. Using the same principle as for the terrace walls, stones are fitted into one another. Of course, a much thicker wall is used for the homes. Each house is two stories high. The upstairs has no windows, but part of the roof is used as a veranda from which to enjoy the view. The floors are connected by a ladder, and the Hunzakuts walk up and down these like acrobats, in perfect balance. The lower floor is occupied in winter. The only heat during these months is supplied by the small fire which is built in the middle of the room. There is a small opening in the ceiling through which the smoke escapes. It connects with the opening in the ceiling of the second floor. This is the only means of ventilation. In summer the family moves upstairs.

One room is used to store food for the winter, and a special place is set aside for food for someone in need during the winter months. "Love thy neighbor as thyself" is demonstrated in its full meaning here.

There is little furniture in the home due to the fact that the majority of the trees that grow in the valley, at one time were imported. Therefore, whatever wood is cut is used only for absolute necessities, such as fuel and building.

In Hunza each man, woman and child responds to the best in himself, the outflow of selflessness. Their philosophy is simple: they have faith in God and believe that He is a partner to all of the children of the universe, and that He has created man to build, to cherish, to love, not to destroy.

Work in Hunza begins at an early hour, five o'clock. Too early, perhaps, for our liking, but there is no kerosene or candles, so they usually retire the moment it grows dark. When the sun slips behind the peaks, the Himalayan moon serves as a lonely beacon in a valley submerged in night. All wood for fires must be preserved for the winter months, when the temperature drops from the average summer temperature of between 80 and 90 degrees to well below zero. Therefore, if the workday is to be well rounded, it must begin as early as possible.

Since there are only two meals served each day, the Hunzakut housewife is spared the task of preparing breakfast. At about noon, the first meal is enjoyed. Food is a vital part of their existence and they eat it for health, not just for its taste, although the latter is generally quite pleasing. Meals are not large and menus do not often vary, but perhaps this is one of the keys to their extraordinary health, as their stomachs are not constantly being overcrammed with superfluous and mineral-sapped foods.

The mainstay of their diet is the chapatti. Although we "educated" Westerners have been cautioned not to eat too much bread, the opposite seems to be true for the Hunzakuts. Of course, the chapattis are made of flour which has not gone through our modern milling processes and is therefore full of nourishing elements.

We must also keep in mind that the manual labor performed by these people daily as they climb the hillsides to their fields causes them to burn up excess carbohydrates much faster than our way of life permits. As a result there are no fat people in Hunza, and also no reducing pills, no gymnastic flab-removing devices and no magic potions that contain "tummy-filling" agents but no calories. In Hunza, no one speaks or thinks of dieting.

7.

Feuds,
Fun
and Games

The Hunzakut language has no word for *boredom*. There is a happy medium between work and play. Hunzakuts often take time off from their work to participate in games or dances; then, when the recreation is over, they return to the fields to finish the work at hand.

One day we were invited to attend and film a game of volleyball. Men from all over the valley had come to Baltit to participate and would be returning to their homes when the game was finished.

The game would pit the "young" men of the valley (sixteen to fifty) against the elders (all over seventy!). The young men included the Mir, his son the Crown Prince, a few teachers from the schools and various villagers. On the team of elders was a man one hundred and twenty-five years young.

Both teams played a strenuous game in the scorching heat of the afternoon sun. If any player was fatigued at any time during the game it was not discernible. They all seemed as relaxed and comfortable as though they were playing a friendly game of canasta.

The winning team claims a sheep from the losing side. Since the state is so small and the grazing land so scarce, there are few sheep in the land. Consequently the value of such an animal is great. After a team wins the prize, there is always a celebration.

The volleyball game was finally over. The team of younger men had won, though only by a few points. When we expressed our amazement at the endurance of the older men, the Mir said with a smile, "When will you people learn that our men of one hundred feel no more fatigue than our men of twenty? And be careful what you say," he jested, "or soon you will have our people of over one hundred feeling three times their age and then they will think they are growing old!"

On that same day we were invited to attend one of the Mir's counsel meetings. I was most anxious to see a Hunzakut court in action, for this is the only country in the world where, although there is no crime, the law is strictly enforced. The Mir and his councilmen meet every day for a court session. The councilmen are the representatives from the various villages, and each serves in the capacity of an elder. Usually an elder dyes his beard with henna which gives him a sign of distinction. These men look quite handsome with their red beards in the morning sun with Mount Rakaposhi as their background.

Each village tries to solve its problems with the help of an elder, who is called an *arbab*. However, as is to be expected, some situations cannot be dealt with without the assistance and advice of the Mir and his council.

They usually meet in front of the new palace, in the patio. They sit on the ground in a semicircle while the Mir sits on a raised podium covered with a Persian rug. Occasionally the court meets on the terrace in front of the old palace, which was built by the Hunzakuts over six hundred years ago. Once the old palace stood as an impregnable fortress. Now it is used only for court sessions or celebrations.

I trudged up the steep mountain road from the playing ground to reach the old palace, which had been chosen for the day's meeting. I was panting and perspiring from the intense heat of the summer sun. Around me moved the people of Hunza. They smiled sympathetically. None of them perspired or panted. They moved quickly at an easy, graceful pace, as though they were moving upward on an escalator. Some of the men had walked all the way to Baltit from as far as 10, 15 or 20 miles away. They would return the same distance and spend the rest of the day working in the fields.

Soon I heard a familiar voice and the Mir and the Crown Prince went gliding past me, the Mir fondly saying as he disappeared over a swell in the road, "See you at the top!" It was most frustrating, but I walked on.

The old palace is three stories high. The court members and the prime minister sat cross-legged on the floor facing the Mir. It was difficult for me to believe, as I watched the court in session, that the Mir holds the power of life and death over his subjects. Open debate was encouraged and if an elder happened to disagree with the Mir he was not afraid to voice his opinion. I soon learned that he was an avid listener and appreciated, as well as hoped to hear, his people's viewpoints on present governmental policies.

It seems that the only friction which ever develops between the Hunzakuts is over such things as irrigation or water rights. All of these frictions, however, are quickly cooled. Each case is put to a vote. The Mir has the final say and can, if he so wishes, veto any decision. But, since he is a wise man, in the majority of cases he goes along with the council's decree. The problem is solved, the decision of how to remedy it accepted and executed. Hunzakuts realize that there is no sense in being stubborn and turning their backs on a decision once it has been made. It stands to reason that the decision rendered is a just one. In Hunza this is well-understood and, after a trial, there are no grievances. Often the two individuals who come to court for a trial will return to their homes together, friends once again.

A few days later the Mir arranged for a polo match, a sport which I have been told originated in Gilgit centuries ago when the armies of Genghis Khan were stationed there. It is said that the Khan's soldiers, bored with an extended period of inactivity, mounted horses and began to bat small rocks around with sticks. Eventually this game grew into the sport we know today, and it has been adopted by almost all of the occupants of the Himalayan regions. However, it was not until the thirteenth century, when Marco Polo came through Hunza on his way from Cathay to India, that the game was to receive a name. Today, polo is the national game of Hunza.

In spite of the shortage of land, each village has set aside a flat piece of ground for polo play. It is carefully preserved and always kept in perfect condition. So, on a beautiful bright afternoon, we all assembled at the Baltit polo grounds to view the game. Seats had been arranged for us on an elevated podium. The fact that I was seated next to the Mir gave me a feeling of comfort, for I had heard rumors about how wild the Hunzakut version of polo could be.

The sky, with the exception of a few delicate fingers of spume blowing from the summit of Mount Rakaposhi, was a subtle yet deep tone of blue. The sun was high and hot, but a fleet of grinning, happy servants stood behind us with umbrellas, which did a fair job of diverting the heat.

On both sides of the field men gathered in their best attire. They sat cross-legged in little groups, looking picturesque among the trees which grew along the entire length of the field. Orchestras were playing, and the unusual tunes of Hunzakut dance music issued enchantingly. Once the game started, however, the music changed and throughout the game drums and flutes beat out a martial tattoo.

Beyond the field, standing on the rooftops, the women were watching. Then, on the field there appeared a young rider, a handsome man seated straight and proud in his saddle. He wore no hat, and in the brilliant sunlight his black hair took on highlights of platinum.

The Mir leaned over to me and said, "This is my nephew. He is an excellent horseman. He is mounted on my personal pet, but I allow him to ride it because he knows how to handle such an animal. In Hunza we have a game of archery which is performed on horseback. He will demonstrate this now and also show you his skill at this game. You see there at the end of the field . . . there where the small pile of earth has been built? Now notice the tiny piece of paper which has been placed in the middle. The rider is expected to pierce that paper with his lance to accomplish his goal."

I watched as the rider gracefully galloped from one end of the field to the other, lowering his lance. He approached his first pass and missed! He tried again, and missed! And still again, and missed! I could hear the impatient murmuring of the crowd below me and turned a questioning gaze to the Mir.

The Mir shook his head with amusement and answered my questioning glances. "The people are most upset with my nephew, I am afraid." He laughed quietly. "They feel his inability to pierce the mark is disgracing the entire state in front of our visitors. They are claiming that there is an eighty-five-year-old youngster among them who can do them honor."

A few moments passed and the eighty-five-year-old "youngster" rose hesitantly, then, spurred on by the applauding crowd, he leaped like a cat to the back of a horse and galloped across the field toward his target. On his first pass he speared the paper. Waving the lance with its prize in the air, he sat in the saddle as tall as possible, his weather-seamed face folded into a true Cheshire-cat grin.

After that, men and horses assembled for polo, all of them lining up in one row, facing the Mir to ask for blessings. The Mir threw the ball and the game was on.

Indeed it was a wild demonstration. The ball flew back and forth. They played vigorously, swinging the polo mallets in all directions and sometimes hitting somebody's head instead of the ball.

Then and there I learned that teeth may be knocked out and bones broken, but the game goes on—and the men won't give up until someone wins. (This explained the toothless grins I had seen here and there.) As there are no dentists in Hunza, the teeth are not replaced. The players who suffer broken bones are more fortunate. There is a bone-setter in every village, and they do a good job. In all my time there, I did not see a single crippled person in Hunza. And, of course, they heal very quickly because of their excellent general health.

Warlike polo is one of the few relics of Hunza's violent past. I sensed the blood of their ferocious ancestors in this almost vicious demonstration, but it lasts only during the game. They play bitterly to the end, hardly obeying any rules. Someone has to win, even if the game lasts for hours. Casualties are accepted as a natural consequence.

The players are wild and reckless. The game is played without rest periods and lasts until one side makes a score of nine goals. Any player who catches a ball in flight can ride through the goal with it, but his opponents are allowed to use any means short of murder to prevent a score.

At this point I noticed that one of the players was bleeding from a deep open wound on his head. Blood covered his face and shirt. But the man didn't seem to mind. He merely took a handkerchief and tied it over the wound as tight as he could, making a sort of a tourniquet, and went on playing to the end.

"Your Highness," I queried, "what happens to the injured?"

"Nothing," he replied, "they just get well."

"What about an infection?"

"Our people seldom get an infection. They rub the wound with some soil rich in minerals and this takes care of any possible infection.

"There are no doctors in Hunza except occasionally foreign medical men come to marvel at our phenomenal freedom from common ills. I have designated a special house to serve as a clinic. They come to us to study and examine our people, I suppose to find the reasons for the outstanding conditions of our older generation. Voluntarily, only a few seek medical advice for minor injuries or similar cases. However, most of them come to me for my miracle salve, a simple salve which I use for everything."

During my stay there was a young Pakistani physician who asked for that assignment to be able to practice in Hunza for a few years.

This was almost unbelievable.

After the game was over the wounded man took part in the dance which is performed by the winning team. He didn't look pale or weak.

The winners bowed gracefully and the game was over—a fabulous demonstration of skill, stamina and perfect health.

8.

The Hunza Way to Live to Be a Hundred

"Birthdays should be happy days, days of thankfulness for being alive and healthy," exclaimed the Mir. "Age has nothing to do with the calendar. Age is simply the ripening of body and mind. Here in Hunza a man's age is reckoned only by his accomplishments: the more he has accomplished, the more wisdom he has acquired, then the greater is his ripeness and value. In this land a man looks forward with happy anticipation to his birthdays."

A slow smile moved on his lips. "I imagine that here it is exactly the opposite to other places. Here the young envy the old and, I am sure that if it were possible, many a young man would try to boost the number of his years so that he might gain a little more respect and admiration from the other youths."

The Mir seemed to read my mind and continued, "In Hunza we have come to know that it is possible to keep pace with time without letting it 'age' us—but then perhaps our entire concept of age differs from yours. You see, we have come to accept the fact that a man's life is divided into three periods: the *young years*, the *middle years* and the *rich years*. In the *young* years there is pleasure and excitement and the yearning for knowledge. In the *middle* years there is the development of poise and appreciation, along with the pleasures, the excitement and the yearnings of the *young* years.

In the *rich* years—by far the best period of all— there is mellowness, understanding, the ability to judge and the great gift of tolerance— all of this combined with the qualities of the two previous periods.

"Indeed, a man in his rich years is truly rich. His life takes on an entirely different scope. It becomes full and completely well rounded. The young people know this and respect this—especially when they see that a man is just as agile mentally and physically as a boy of twenty.

"So you see, my sister, our viewpoints on this subject differ somewhat. From the day a Hunzakut is born, he is never coddled. He keeps active until the day he dies, and does not think about growing old. Here there is time to think only of the necessary things. To worry over such an intangible thing as the ticking of a clock, or the turning of a page on a calendar, this is foolishness."

"But the elder members of your society—the men and women over ninety—don't they ever retire from work?" I asked.

Again there was that slow smile. "The idleness of retirement is a much greater enemy to life than work. One must never retire 'from' something. One must retire 'to' something. Our people continue to work on by choice."

He paused momentarily, then added, "You know, it has been always my contention that a man is very much like a plant. He must have a very strong sense of belonging, otherwise he will wither and die, just as a plant will die if it is placed in an alien and infertile soil. To take a man or woman, simply because they have reached a certain age, and put them in some 'resting' place away from all contact with their functioning society, this is the same as a death warrant.

"I go abroad," the Mir continued, "and meet people of other countries, of other races. I can detect a feeling of restlessness and tension in most of them. The ability to relax is at the bottom of everything. Watch the Hunza people at work or at rest. They are completely relaxed, completely at ease. For instance, watch our royal cook sit for hours in a squatting position on the floor baking chapattis—at ninety years of age her hands are strong and young.

"Cheerfulness is the best mental tonic. Enjoyment is already part of our battle. If you enjoy your work, you will do it in a relaxed manner, while hate and grumbling will create tension and the nerves will become jumpy. Don't you know that we are the mirror of our thoughts?"

"If this is so," I said, "then the mind controls the body, especially the nervous system."

"Practically, although it can be said to work the other way too, at which time the body influences the mind. There is no doubt that the body and the mind are bound together and must function in a complete balance. A pain in some part of the body will cause a mental depression."

"If your theory is correct, your people have achieved a complete control over body and mind, and can control their pains, too. I observed them many times at their various occupations, as well as during meditation, and I could sense their complete inner peace."

"As an example," the Mir said, "if some of my people get injured, cut or burn themselves, they would come to me for help. I have a salve which I apply to the injured spot, and the person goes away with a conviction that he is healed. Confidence and control over his body are responsible for it. I have been using the same salve for everything. You know very well that it is not the medication that releases the pain.

"Remember the man who was injured so badly while playing polo? He didn't get any infection. The good earth applied to his wound took care of this. We well know that a man requires medication or treatment when his body is sick. But our men don't get ill, because they control their nerves, their whole system, by sensible living.

"My people work slowly, without any great rush which, according to your Western pattern of doing things, would seem a lazy way, and some would wonder whether they accomplish anything. However, I can assure you that they do accomplish a great deal during each day, and by all means they couldn't be considered a lazy people. Some people mistake laziness for a relaxed attitude."

"No, Mir Sahib! No, your people are by no means lazy. I remember on the trail as I was coming, their stamina was amazing. I admired them for their good disposition. No matter how hard some of the old men worked repairing the road in the terrible heat, they always smiled."

"This is correct," the Mir's eyes were shining with pride. "My people have a reputation all over the Himalayan region to be excellent workers, willing to accept the most difficult assignment. Nothing can stop us. If a job has to be done, it is done!

"The political agent of Gilgit, Rehman Khan, has encouraged

some of my people to move to Gilgit. He offered them land to settle down there. Since we are being overpopulated and are so short of land, some were obliged to move, although, as you know, they leave Hunza reluctantly. The land they got in Gilgit was an undeveloped terrain and hardly suitable for agricultural needs; nevertheless, in a short time they turned this land into beautiful fields with fine crops. They are hard workers and love their work.

"Here, where we must work hard to exist, we cannot waste any energy and it is very clear that anyone who doesn't understand or doesn't practice the techniques of relaxation is wasting a great deal of energy. The individual who is capable of relaxing will enjoy vitality and endurance and will accomplish his job faster than the person who works under tension. The body and mind are intimately connected and function together.

"To explain better what I mean, watch a Hunzakut, whether man or woman, or even a child. He takes a rest in between work even if only for a few minutes. He sits down in a comfortable position. His every muscle and nerve is relaxed, and he remains silent for as long as he chooses to be. He prays in the same position twice a day, and rests in between work. You have seen Hunzakuts sitting in the middle of the street oblivious to outside activities when resting or meditating. It takes training of the mind to be able to concentrate in noisy surroundings!

"The ability to relax every muscle and nerve in our body, even for a few minutes, protects the muscles from overwork. Thus my men can walk for miles and then return to work in the fields without a sign of fatigue. They know the secrets of relaxation."

The Mir was right. Many times, while walking through the streets of Baltit, I had seen people sitting cross-legged on the ground, eyes closed, oblivious to the outside world. I quietly passed them, not to disturb their mood. In fact, once I saw a child of about six years sitting next to an older man, maybe his father, in exactly the same position. The child's eyes were closed, and there was a radiant smile on his face.

Somewhere in the onrush of civilization, man acquired a notion that he must accumulate possessions by pushing and driving himself to a frenzy. In the process of doing so, man lost the ability to replenish his inner power, and consequently he undergoes great strain, which is wearing out his bodily strength and resistance.

Then we feed our bodies with food lacking in nourishment. We have no time to sit down to relax for a few minutes or be silent. We have no time to take a daily walk or exercise. Nervous tension shortens our lives. A man easily irritated cannot have complete peace of mind because his nerves, muscles and brain are constantly under high tension.

The Mir said, "There is no need for the body to get sick under the strain of life or for the mind to shatter under tension or the heart to fail because it is driven beyond its strength."

Suddenly it was clear to me that these people possess that elusive secret of happiness which might be the key to the fountain of youth. Without education or books, they have acquired the greatest knowledge of all—the knowledge of relaxation, peace of mind and long life.

If only we all could realize and remember this, how much better our tomorrows might be. Right now is a good time to take an inventory of our health, our thoughts, of our environment, of the persons with whom we work and of the work we do, and carefully analyze our actions. We, too, can design a perfect life acceptable to everyone's taste. "An open mind is the fount of eternal youth."

I was indebted to the Mir for this conversation. It cleared my mind considerably. What a great thinker he was and what a great soul! How fortunate I was to know him and be adopted by him and his family and inherit the title of "sister."

"The idleness of retirement is a much greater enemy to life than work." Those were the words he had used. I got out of bed and stood by the window. A bright moon, shining on the icy sides of Mount Rakaposhi, bathed the entire valley in an ethereal glow of sufficient brightness for me to identify whitewashed houses miles away. No light was visible and the place seemed to be an unpopulated portion of another world. For a moment I took the bright moon for daybreak.

Quietly I slipped out of the house. Silence was absolute; no dogs barking, no squealing brakes, no honking horns. The air was pleasant and cool. The weather can be compared to California's. The nights are always cool and fresh, even if the day's temperature gets as high as 100 or over. And in the daytime there is always a cool breeze from the mountains.

I realized that these towering mountains had protected this tiny valley for over 2,000 years, preserving a civilization from the rest of the world, permitting the development of a hardy people of unparalleled lifespan.

Perhaps, aside from the magnificent nutrition of the Hunzakuts, their mental attitude was the key to their extraordinary longevity. Until a few years ago, many scientists believed that all living things had a fixed "clock" ticking away and dictating the limits of their lifespans. But recent experiments and the very existence of the Hunzakuts have proved this to be incorrect.

Could it be that age is predominantly a state of mind? Is it possible that the secret of life lies in a psychic concept rather than a physical one? Is it possible for, let us say, an American man of eighty with the proper attitude toward life to take vigorous morning horseback rides, play three or four sets of tennis on a hot day, go camping in the High Sierras or try his hand at surfing at Waikiki with as much ease and proficiency as a boy of twenty? Could he do all this with only the aid of a sound diet and a sound state of mind? Or was it true that, once the human body reaches a certain point, it begins to deteriorate?

"The idleness of retirement is a much greater enemy to life than work." Again the Mir's words stirred in my mind. How many people had I known who had literally been forced into retirement? Many! A few had chosen retirement, but the majority of them had simply reached a certain age and were, as a result, relieved of their work. I had often listened to their complaints, but had never, until this moment, really given the matter much thought.

Age should have nothing to do with the retirement plan. If a man is mentally and physically able to work, and wants to do so, why should he be callously dropped into the realm of unending shuffleboard matches, bridge games, mineral baths and the frustrations of not being able to contribute to his society simply because he is chronologically a month or two older than what has been accepted as the "proper" working age? Without initiative and the knowledge that an elderly person is an integral part of his community, there is only one end—slow stagnation of the spirit. Once the spirit of an individual rots away, the body begins to lose its incentive to produce strong muscles, bones, tissues and cells until one day some small part of the complex human mechanism simply ceases to function and death becomes an easy victor.

That was what the Mir had meant. In Hunza there was no retirement. In Hunza that lonely angel called "death" never won an easy victory.

This brought me to the inevitable question I am always asked: "What is the point of living an amazingly long life?" Does a Hunzakut woman enjoy her longevity? Is it possible that she never complains about her endless making of chapattis and apricot oil? Does she never weary of walking to the river to bathe or wash her laundry? Does she ever feel the pangs of remorse at not participating in the games and festivities which so color the lives of the men of Hunza? Does she feel no resentment for her lack of education?

Does a Hunzakut man enjoy his longevity? Is it possible that he never complains about his endless toil in the fields? Does he never, as he sees the men and women from beyond the mountains, wonder what lies beyond the mystic ranges of the Korakorum and the Himalaya? Does he feel no sense of inadequacy when met by well-educated Westerners?

My thoughts were interrupted by a piercing chant. Sounds like *ommmomommmm* found their echo beyond the impregnable mountain walls. It was like a voice from heaven calling to the people on earth.

On my first day in Hunza, when this voice woke me up at the dim light of daybreak, I thought someone was serenading me. But when I saw no one in front of my window, I went back to sleep. And not until I questioned the Mir about it did I learn that every morning at 3:30 A.M. in summer the prayer man calls the Hunza-kuts to get up to pray before they begin their work; and in the evening, as the sun goes down, he calls them to pray before they retire.

Since there is no electricity, no kerosene, and no candles, the people of Hunza are obliged to retire early and rise early. They have happily accepted their way of life.

With the last note of the chant, the mysterious quietness took its grip again. Such peace and beauty! People began to move out of their homes without making any noise, as though they were afraid to disturb the silence which lay over the valley. Some went toward the little mosque, built in every village, where they met for prayers; some sat down in front of their homes, or on their open balcony on the second floor—all of them were equally engulfed in deep meditation.

I, too, prayed in quiet meditation. A gay voice brought me back to reality. "*Salaam*, Missy!" It was one of the young Hunzakuts whom I knew. He was a man of about twenty-three, married and a proud father of a five-year-old boy. "Good morning, Ullah," I replied.

"You are up before the sun," he said.

I could not help but admire his fine pronunciation of the English tongue which he learned in school in Rawalpindi. I felt like asking him the questions I had just asked myself, for he had witnessed life outside this community. He would not be governed by prejudices. When I had finished, he stared somberly across the village out to where the first rays of dawn were beginning to color the pinnacle of Mount Rakaposhi, making the mountain seem as though it were blushing at the thought of being seen in its naked splendor.

"The questions you ask are good questions," he replied. "But you see, my people are not like people from beyond the mountains. When I was in the Pakistani school and then in the army, I learned this very quickly. My people know very little discontent. We have a great love for our way of life. We do not question it."

"But don't you ever want to better things for yourself and your family?"

He nodded. "Yes, I do. But the way we live is the way of my fathers. I will change it a little as I learn better ways, just as my sons will change it a little after I have left them. It is a good way to be. We ask nothing of anyone. What we learn, we learn in our own time, and this is good. It is exciting to know that our knowledge has been discovered by us: the way to make the fields fertile and rich with promise; the way to make the barren mountainsides burst into life with wheat and corn and growing things of many kinds and colors; the way to make music echo up to the glaciers; the way to make light and fires that do not smoke too much; the way to raise our cattle; the way to tease the melting snows and make them work for us and give us food; the way to make flour and chapattis. All of these things we have learned—by our own efforts. We are proud of this. It is a good way. No one wants to leave this place. Banishment from this land is the greatest punishment for any of us.

"In other places," he continued, "men hurry from one task to another. While they work at one thing, they are already worrying what their next job will be. I do not understand this. Here in Hunza each task is done with love. A man is lucky to have a field to work. He is lucky to be able to feel the warm sun and know that his muscles move in rhythm with his work. He is lucky to be able to see the beauty which lies all around him. A man is surely blessed to be born into this life, to be given the strength and ability to work his land and raise his family, to laugh and to sing and to know the cold of winter and the joy of spring."

As Ullah walked away, I realized that a Hunzakut has learned to accept his life and to live it fully. He tolerates privation and hardship in winter because he knows that this will make him doubly appreciate the abundance and beauty of spring. He tolerates the oppressive heat of summer because he knows how well he will look forward to the cool winds of autumn.

As I strolled along the narrow streets, villagers on their way to the field passed me with a friendly smile and with the usual greeting, "*Salaam*." I returned the greetings in the same fashion. What contented and happy faces, I thought, echoers of that spirit and peace of mind.

On a stone bench next to one of the homes, an older man was holding a baby. Since men here father children at eighty and ninety, it very well could have been his son. I stopped. This man looked like a wise old soul, and I wanted to talk to him. Maybe he, too, spoke English, and would be able to answer some of my questions.

After exchanging greetings he motioned for me to sit down next to him. The old man looked at me with a friendly smile. His black eyes were shining with a light of a youth. A thick head of black hair and the smooth skin on his face were all indications of a young man, but possibly, according to his calendar age he wasn't a young man anymore. The baby was the image of him. He was indeed the father!

I admired both of them and could not help but ask, "How old are you?" We in the Western world are so conscious of our age that it is one of the first questions we are asked when we meet a new acquaintance or when we apply for a job. From earliest childhood, age is a topic invariably discussed everywhere—among old and young alike—and dreaded as poison.

"Missy," he replied, "my age is none of my business!" His English was a pleasant surprise. "The number of years we live is unimportant." He spoke slowly to make sure that his English would be understood. "The kind of years we live is important. Eternal life is a quality of life, not a quantity. A man of eighty can be young while a man of thirty can be old."

His philosophy was astounding. He looked about fifty, but he told me that he was about eighty.

The baby sat quietly, smiling. Children behave so well in Hunza, and in the presence of adults they listen attentively, as if they understood the meaning of the conversation.

"To think about age is to become a slave to it," continued my wise stranger. "Why should we consider adding twenty-four hours to our bodies because the earth has made another revolution in its eternal path around the sun? No one can determine your age unless you tell them. If man could live without clocks and calendars he would be better off! We here determine time by the sun and stars, and the sky, so how can a number of days influence our age?"

There was so much vigor and life in this man. And so much wisdom—natural wisdom and common sense. I wanted to hear more, so I sat patiently and encouraged him to go on talking.

"The true keynote of life is growth, not aging. Life does not grow old. The life that flows through us at eighty is the same that energized us in infancy. It does not get old or weak. So-called age is the deterioration of enthusiasm, faith to live, and the will to progress. I am eighty years old! I don't feel any different now from when I was twenty or forty. No one here ever talks of age, or even mentions that he or she is too old to do things, and surely you are never too old to be happy to be alive. I went to school in Gilgit, and I learned from your big books, but our people here, the majority anyway, learn from nature, and they know what is good for them."

Western scientists are now agreeing that early aging is unnecessary and that every person should be able to renew his youth and vigor in cases where disease is not already present. It is now a well-known fact that our body cells are continually being renewed. It was once thought that complete renewal occurred only every seven years, but now we are told that certain cells are renewed in a matter of months. Our bodies are continuously in the process of casting off worn-out cells and replacing them with new ones.

If this is true, then all men can take advantage of it. We should eat well to begin with so that as new cells are born they will be healthy and strong. In time our bodies will be rejuvenated. We should exercise our bodies and minds and control our emotions.

We grow old because we believe we must. Nature produces the body cells and we stamp them with our habits of thought, making them something nature never intended them to be. It is amazing to note how little interest mankind has taken in investigating the actual cause of cell deterioration.

Life is a perpetual process of tearing down and building up. Potentially it has perfect balance, but human ignorance and error have interfered with its rhythmic equilibrium. Our body has an inherent, automatic and practically unlimited power of renewal. If we regard life as something eternal and indestructible, it should be possible to remain both mentally young and physically fit indefinitely.

Growing old, even gracefully, has gone out of fashion. Dr. Joseph W. Still of George Washington University, Washington, D.C., says, "Aging is simply a disease."

And Dr. Henry S. Simms of Columbia University, New York City, one of the top experts on aging, estimates that "if a person remained as healthy as he is when he is fifteen or twenty years old, he would live for hundreds of years." By this he means that the lifespan of any creature depends on how fast its body cells mature.

Dr. Lord Taylor, one of England's leading physicians, told the House of Lords in London in December of 1961, "If people can avoid all the diseases of the heart and blood vessels, there seems to be no particular reason why they should die at all."

If this is true, wouldn't it prove the Hunza theory—that death is decided by choice!

The Russians are also looking for the secrets of eternal life. One of their top scientists, Vladimir T. Kuprevich, said, "Why should man die of old age? I consider the process of aging an abnormal process. I am sure we can find means for switching off the mechanism which makes cells age. Then man, his body cells eternally renewed as they aged, would become immortal. Scientists the world over believe that their eternal-life experiments are leading to a revolution far greater in its potential significance than the atomic or hydrogen bombs."

Each of our cells has a specific job to do, and it must have the proper nutrients if it is to do the job effectively. As the cells wear out they are replaced by others and, if proper nourishment is provided, the new cells retain the healthy qualities of the old. The bodies of many people start to deteriorate in middle life because their diets lack proteins, vitamins and minerals—especially proteins.

The composition of a person's body depends on what he eats. Food is anything which, when digested, furnishes the material that the cells need to keep their structure healthy and their functions normal. As long as we feed our cells with a balanced diet, providing the essential materials such as oxygen, water, carbohydrates, proteins, vitamins, enzymes and inorganic elements, we will keep them alive and full of vigor. Then there would be no reason to age.

The quality of food plays an important part in providing body-building essentials. Hunza gardens and fields grow nourishing produce because their soil is so rich in organic elements.

People as a rule pay little attention to their health until they lose it. We must use our common sense, just as the Hunzakuts do, and make it a daily practice to eat properly and live sensibly.

We must realize that a balanced, natural diet will supply us with the necessary proteins, vitamins and minerals our bodies need. If we all lived in Hunza we wouldn't need to be so concerned. But in the rest of the world, where so much artificiality has been incorporated into our way of living, we must be sure where our food comes from in order to secure that necessary balance. Therefore, to fortify our bodies with a dependable, balanced food supplement in tablets or capsules is important. However, we must know how to take these supplements, as they should also be considered as food and should be balanced with our diet. Therefore, a careful study of nutrition is just as important as learning to read and write. We must pay a great price for ignorance.

Obesity is another dominating factor to good health. Keep your weight down and do not eat too much. Your body cannot carry an excess amount of fat and get away with it. Besides, fat can only cause you trouble. By eating sensibly you will not need to worry about these additional pounds. You should always weigh the same! You don't need to increase your measurements because you have added a few years to your body. Continue to be active and you will experience no change.

I have given you the secrets of the marvelous people of Hunza, of people who are probably vaguely aware of their sensible habits. I have written of their attitude toward life, their approach to hardships and dangers, to worry and drudgery. All of this indicates that they have found the secret—if not of eternal life—to a life rich with at least a hundred exciting, beautiful and rewarding years.

You, too, can drink at the same Fountain of Youth.

By now the village was wide awake and everyone was at work. The ancient castle which was built by the Mir's ancestors stood there high in all its morning glory. I looked up and marvelled at its structure. For 600 years it had withstood all kinds of weather!

Suddenly I felt someone was staring at me. It was my friend, a 145-year youngster. He didn't speak a word of English, but he had a happy smile, and when he looked at me, I felt I knew what he was saying. He remembered some wonderful tales and stories that he would tell the children, and they in turn would tell others. His long white beard was soft and his white hair beautifully thick and well kept. Tall and slim he looked so youthful in the bright sun.

We exchanged our greetings, our smiles, and since we could not speak to each other, I followed him down the winding trail. His graceful walk and straight posture made me conscious of my own —I pulled up my shoulders. He proudly led me to the playing grounds where the Mir himself was playing a game of volley-ball with some of his elders. The majority of the elders looked to me to be fifty or maybe sixty; however, I knew they were much older. My 145-year old friend joined the group and got into the act. When I saw him jumping up to catch the ball, just as a young lad, I hardly could believe my own eyes. But, after you have lived with these people, you get used to miracles.

After the game was over, I watched the men disappear toward the old castle—1200 feet up the hill—to meet with the Mir in their daily court session. Since women aren't supposed to be present, I remained behind, admiring the group climbing up the steep road. Although the Mir had invited me many times to join him in court, I didn't want to break their customary rules and be different from their women.

Instead I visited the schoolhouse. As I entered the room, the boys got up and shouted in English, "Good morning!" The teacher was explaining English grammar! Here thousands of miles away, children were learning our English language. It was a pleasant thought! I shall never forget their young faces shining with delight and joy and their sparkling eyes as they sat silently and listened to the teacher with a glowing acceptance of what they heard.

Children here are treated with courtesy and they return the same. The grown-ups seem to be aware that children learn from what they encounter in the world around them. We teach our children to behave, to obey, to have good manners, and then the adults so often aren't able to control their emotions in front of them. I remember an embarrassing moment, when a son of one of my dear friends once told me, after he listened to a quarrel of his parents—"Manners seem to be for children only!"

Not far off, men were occupied with threshing. With the hooves of the animals the grain is separated from the chaff, to be stored for future use. A group of animals—mules and cows—were led by men round and round a small field where the grain was spread.

The canal, filled with the rich mineral water winding its way through the village and providing water for irrigation and domestic use looked cool and inviting. The grey color gave it a "pearlized" appearance. Because of its color, the Hunzakuts refer to it as "our glacial milk." Everyone drinks an abundance of this water which is not boiled or filtered. Even the children enjoy this water and you see them drinking it all the time directly from the streams. These people are indeed geniuses in concocting things for their comfort without tools or mechanical devices. Some of the scientists who have analyzed their water, and found it rich in minerals, have suggested that the water might be responsible for their excellent health. Our bodies require minerals in great quantities and this water is full of them.

Following the stream, I reached the village community mill. Here the head miller was preoccupied with making fresh flour. The water supplied the power for his primitive hand-stone grist mill. The fine flour was spread all around the stone, and the man was collecting it in one pile. He gave me a handful of whole wheat grain in, I assume, a gesture of friendliness.

I learned that he also was the head weaver; and as soon as he finished his morning job of preparing the flour for the villagers, he took a seat at the handmade loom in the same cottage. He worked for the rest of the day weaving the necessary fabrics for winter clothing. The sheep supplied the wool from which he made lovely soft coats. This man owned no land. The generous farmers supplied him and his family with sufficient food for the whole year. His time was devoted to crafts.

Baking was done in a specially built cottage on the palace

grounds. "Nanie," the royal baker, sitting on the floor, her feet under her body, was kneading the dough for the bread on a low table in front of her. She was a master cook and no wonder—for seventy years she had been baking chapattis and other goodies for the palace household. After all there were a hundred mouths to feed, and now there were seven more of us.

Her hands moved fast and gracefully. They were strong hands, young hands. But I knew she was almost 90 years old. The native dress, the spotlessly white pantaloons, the red sheath long blouse, and the colorful pillbox hat looked so dainty with this simple background. Two long black braids hung loose on both sides of her radiant face. White teeth sparkled through the well-shaped mouth which was not touched by lipstick. And there were no other traces of magic beauty potions. Although her skin was clean, healthy looking and very smooth, I suppose apricot oil was doing the trick, or the fresh air, or the good food, or her cheerful disposition—a combination of everything!

Her assistant, in her seventies, dressed alike, with a delightful smile was handing things to her superior to make it easier for her. The little room, which hardly could be called a room, had a fire built in the middle—covered with a thin grill on which the chapattis were baked, a small table, and a cupboard. Both women looked slim and graceful. They projected contentment.

There is something about these people that unfolds an intimacy of friendliness assuring you of your welcome. There is something else worthy of mentioning: You always hear music. Whether they play games, work, rest, or exercise, someone is always playing tunes of melodious quality inviting everyone to hum or to dance. The sounds of the drum and the flute softly sweep through the air.

The magic of the summer morning was in the air. The smell of flowers permeated the quiet garden—an oasis of green lawns, flowers, and fruit trees in this spectacular setting of Himalayan splendor.

The Crown Prince Ghazanfar was playing a game of tennis with a friend. Skillfully handling the ball, he obviously was not a novice. The whole royal family enjoys tennis, and there is a spacious court built in the garden.

From below, occasional voices broke the silence of the garden. Some youngsters were playing in the ice cold water of the swimming pool. These two modern facilities in this most remote spot of the world made me wonder!

I looked for Princess Azra, the youngest daughter, then only eight years old and beautiful. The cherry tree was our secret spot to meet early in the morning to pick the fruit directly from the tree, but she wasn't there. It was later than usual and she must have gone indoors. The Princesses, Fauzia 14 years old, Mehr Ul Jamal 15, Malika Hussn 16, Nilofar 19, and Duri Shahwar 22, including Princess Azra, were all studying with the English governess Mrs. Hansen. She conducted regular daily classes on a level of our high school, and the girls as a rule spent all morning in class. They were very conscientious about their work and were eager to learn. Even the Queen studied with Mrs. Hansen in order to perfect her English. Prince Ghazanfar Ali Khan, Prince Amen Khan, and Prince Abbas Khan attended English boarding schools in Rawalpindi.

The cherries were hanging low and easy to reach. Every branch was covered with fruit and no matter how many were picked, the fruit didn't seem to diminish. Each cherry was juicy and sweet—not a single one eaten by a worm. My eyes caught other trees, and every one was covered with beautiful fruit—apples, pears of enormous size—a pound each. The peaches and apricots were luscious and juicy, and the grapes grew in abundance on huge trees. Women were picking grapes to make vinegar and the famous Hunza wine.

In Hunza, after trees grow for fifty years, the tops are cut off, and the trees continue to bring fruit—an indication that the soil is rich and healthy.

Completely captured by the spell of the whole valley, the friendly, kind and joyous people, the snow capped peaks, the garden with its exotic flower arrangements, and the music mixed with the sweet murmur of the wind, I saw everything in a new light. Why can't we learn that the readiness to enjoy life is no shallow childishness but the deep source of blessed living?

"Good morning," came a voice from nowhere and broke my spell. Her Highness was nursing her flowers. There was a rich variety of them—all in bloom—the same flowers you find in our gardens in sunny California.

Finding the Rani in the midst of all this was like finding a shining candle amidst the lovely colors. She loves nature, colors, the flowing of the life force that is in everything formed by creation. This garden is her shrine!

She seems so delicate, but as you know her better and watch her function, you begin to feel the boundless strength of an eternal energy. She keeps busy all day long as do all the other women of Hunza. She manages her household—over one hundred people who have to be clothed, fed, and all their needs taken care of. She also counsels the women who come to her for advice daily. She is a great help to her husband and always has the time to be with her children in the afternoon. Indeed, her day is well planned.

She was coming toward me. "We missed you at breakfast!" she said in a simple way, "and I know that we'll miss you when you leave us!" I knew she was sincere and I also knew that I had found a new friend.

She took me by the arm and said: "But then what is time in comparison with eternity? You will be back! Anyone who understands us and loves our land the way you do, will be back! Maybe then, you will stay here longer! And now, run along, I must return to my duties!"

Deeply impressed by her simplicity and humbleness, tears formed in the corners of my eyes, and I held back the urge to start crying. The friendliness of this land seemed to reach out and enfold me at that moment. Which is greater, worldly wealth that is here today and gone tomorrow or the wealth of divine love that God has stored upon these people? Divine love is the magnet that draws all good! The wealth of divine love has met every need of man!

9.

The Amazing
Hunza Diet

Over fifty years ago, Dr. Robert McCarrison, a brilliant English surgeon, took up the study of certain diseases common to the peoples of Asia.

He was interested in finding out to what degree diseases in Indian peoples were caused by faulty food. He wrote in his book *Studies in Deficiency Diseases*:

> My own experience provides an example of a race unsurpassed in perfection of physique and in freedom from disease in general. I refer to the people of the State of Hunza, situated in the extreme northernmost point of India. . . . Amongst these people the span of life is extraordinarily long; and such service as I was able to render them during the seven years I spent in their midst was confined chiefly to the treatment of accidental lesions, the removal of senile cataract, plastic operations for granular lids, or the treatment of maladies wholly unconnected with food supply.
>
> During the period of my association with these people, I never saw a case of asthenic dyspepsia, of gastric or duodenal ulcer, or appendicitis, of mucous colitis, or cancer. . . . Among these people the "abdomen oversensitive" to nerve impressions, to fatigue, anxiety or cold was unknown. The

consciousness of the existence of this part of their anatomy was, as a rule, related solely to the feeling of hunger. Indeed, their buoyant abdominal health has, since my return to the West, provided abdominal contrast with the dyspeptic and colonic lamentations of our highly civilized communities.

Dr. McCarrison found that the Pathans, who live in the region of the Khyber Pass, were great hillsmen and adept at primitive agriculture. They ate comparatively well and were by no means a lazy people. The Sikhs also fit into this category. In an article written by him in 1925, Dr. McCarrison wrote that the Sikhs, the Pathans and certain other Himalayan tribes "are of fine physical development and power of endurance, but by no means even compare with the Hunzakuts."

The question that now absorbed his mind was: "How is it that man can be such a magnificent physical creature as the Hunzakut?" And he proceeded to view the ills of both civilized and uncivilized man.

In 1927, Dr. McCarrison was appointed Director of Nutrition Research in India under the Research Fund Association.

For his work and experiments he chose albino rats. Rats are largely used in nutritional laboratories because they love all human food. Their span of life is short, so their whole life history can be observed.

For the first phase of his experiment, Dr. McCarrison chose healthy rats, then placed them in good conditions, with fresh air, sunlight, comfort and cleanliness. He chose their diet from foods eaten regularly by the Hunzakuts: chapattis made of wholemeal flour, lightly smeared with fresh butter; sprouted pulse; fresh raw carrots; raw cabbage; unboiled milk; a small ration of meat with bones once a week, and an abundance of water.

In this experiment almost 1,200 rats were watched from birth to the twenty-seventh month, an age in the rat which corresponds to that of about fifty years in a man. At this stage the Hunza-diet-fed rats were killed and carefully examined. McCarrison's report was remarkable:

> During the past two and a quarter years there has been no case of illness in this "universe" of albino rats, no death from natural causes in the adult stock, and, but for a few accidental deaths, no infantile mortality. Both clinically and at

postmortem, examination of this stock has been shown to be remarkably free from disease. It may be that some of them have cryptic disease of one kind or another, but if so, I have failed to find either clinical or microscopical evidence of it.

His experiments did not, however, stop here. Next he took *diseased* rats and placed them, too, on the Hunzakut diet. They all became well. Then he took batches of rats and placed them in clean, comfortable surroundings and fed them the food of the people of India. The rats living on the various Indian diets, which consisted of rice, pulses, cooked vegetables and condiments were soon plagued with diseases and miseries of many kinds. Over two thousand rats fed on faulty Indian diets developed eye ailments, ulcers, boils, bad teeth, crooked spines, loss of hair, anemia, skin disorders, heart, kidney and glandular weaknesses and a multitude of gastrointestinal disorders.

In later experiments, McCarrison gave a set of rats the diet of the poorer classes of England: white bread, margarine, sweetened tea, boiled vegetables, tinned meats and inexpensive jams and jellies. On this diet, not only did the rats develop all kinds of disease conditions, but they became nervous wrecks: "They were nervous and apt to bite their attendants; they lived unhappily together, and by the sixteenth day of the experiment they began to kill and eat the weaker ones amongst them."

Hunzakuts eat mainly grain (including wheat, barley, buckwheat and small grains); leafy green vegetables; potatoes and other root vegetables; peas and beans; gram of chick pea and other pulses; fresh milk and buttermilk, or *lassi*; clarified butter and cheese; fruit, chiefly apricots and mulberries, fresh and sun-dried; meat on rare occasions, and wine made from grapes.

Let's analyze the nutritional values of each product and see why the Hunzakuts have chosen these particular foods for their diet.

Of cereal foods and bread, they eat wheat and a great deal of millet. Sometimes a chick pea is ground up with the wheat, sometimes beans, barley and peas are all mixed together and ground into flour, from which they make a flat bread called chapatti. The grinding is also different. The whole grain remains in the flour and as a result is very nourishing. We usually grind our grain to a fine white powder and in most cases discard the valuable nutrients.

BREAD (Chapatti)

The Hunza bread is wholesome, unrefined, maybe even coarse, but full of good nourishment. During pioneer days in America, grain was stoneground in small quantities just as the need arose for the day, but then the increase in population forced nutrition experts to invent other means and large mills were erected to produce flour in large quantities.

The part of the grain from which the new plant grows is called the germ. This germ is actually the most nourishing portion of the grain, but since it is oily it tends to become rancid very quickly and therefore is not left in most commercial flour, which is to be stored, as it would cause spoilage. It is all crushed with the help of large steel rollers. Then the germ is sifted out to separate it from the flour, allowing only the white, starchy part to be used by the public.

The outer covering of the grain is known as bran. In the commercial processing, or milling, of grain this bran is also removed. When it is left in, it gives the flour a brownish overtone. People have become accustomed to associate the quality of the flour with the purity of color and consequently choose the white flour in preference to the dark. The main objective of commercial flour is that it must have a long shelf life so it won't spoil or attract insects.

The wheat germ, which supplies Vitamin E, is also the part of the grain which seems to assist the sexual powers of an animal who eats it. It invigorates the whole animal through the strengthening of the reproductive system, as well as the whole glandular system and special organs such as the heart and general muscular condition. An experiment conducted by H. A. Mattill, M.D. and reported in the *American Journal of Physiology*, as far back as 1927, indicates that vitamin E which is found in the wheat germ kernel, plays an important part in the reproductive powers of the animal. Dr. Evan Shute of Canada, whose work with vitamin E and heart disease is famous, reports in the *Urological and Cutaneous Review*, Volume 48, 1944, using vitamin E extensively in therapy for reproductive disorders.

Hunza bread consists of all of the nutrients of the grain. Perhaps this accounts for their strong nerves and vigor into old age, for they eat plenty of bread with every meal. This may account for the fact that the men of ninety are capable of fathering children and the women able to conceive at fifty years of age.

Someone has aptly said, "The taste for white flour, polished white rice and white sugar is an illustration of the failure of the instinct of man to serve as a safe guide in the selection of foods."

It is possible that man has progressed too fast, and in the process lost all instinct, or so-called common sense, regarding his diet.

Naturally, our modern loaf of white bread is enriched artificially. But why destroy the natural goodness of the grain and then replace it artificially? It seems a little silly when you stop to think about it. And why must we have white bread? To get that loaf of white bread the wheat has to be milled and treated in a manner that destroys the natural source of nourishment.

The people of Hunza have never eaten white bread. Having lived for generations on the sturdy brown bread of their chapatti, they would not find white bread appetizing. On one occasion during the trip we tried to feed our drivers spaghetti made of white flour, but they refused to eat it. Surely the white color did not perk up their appetites. They thought that such a soft mass should be fed to people without teeth.

The chapatti, which is the mainstay of their diet, is made from wheat, barley, buckwheat or millet flour. It is rich in phosphorus, potassium, iron, calcium, manganese and other minerals, as nothing has been destroyed in the preparation of the flour from the wheat. Thus the chapatti contains the essential nourishment of the grain.

Usually prepared in several shapes, small or large, they are baked on top of a grill, built over an open low fire. To make a good tasty chapatti, the flour has to be freshly ground, including the bran, then the dough kneaded to a right consistency (and only an experienced hand can determine the "right consistency") so the chapatti won't be tough. To obtain the desired quality the flour, the dough and the preparation of it will be responsible for its taste. The recipe is simple and everyone from childhood on—boys and girls—are taught how to make chapattis.

During our trip, whenever we stopped for a rest, our drivers prepared chapattis for their meal. They carried their small handmill along and a sack of wheat, and made fresh flour for the bread, which they baked over an open fire. Proper food means existence, and not a single Hunzakut will chance his health. Wherever he goes, his healthful eating habits are observed. He will never leave home without a supply of his own grain and a handmill.

The chapatti has a taste that is very satisfying; it is chewy and exercises the gums. A piece of it together with a few apricots is a complete meal for a Hunzakut, along with a few glasses of their cooling "glacial milk." They certainly seem to thrive on this frugal diet. Everyone is sturdy and full of energy, especially the old men.

MILK

Milk is considered a complete food. In Hunza it is used in various ways. First the cream is separated from the milk to make *ghee*. It is simply left at room temperature, and when it thickens it is ready to be eaten. It tastes very good, and I have hardly noticed the difference from our regular butter. Cottage cheese is made from the remains, a vital source of protein in their diet.

Such things as butter, milk and cheese, made mostly from goat's milk, are delicacies. In the higher regions of the valley, where goats and cows do not fare well, the yak is a source of dairy products and also serves as a means of transportation and labor.

The buttermilk, or *lassi*, that is left is drunk with their meals. Yogurt is very popular. They usually sour milk, and even sour buttermilk, as it keeps much better when soured. There is no refrigeration, so they have to use their imaginations to protect food from spoilage. In a country which has a limited amount of food, it is essential to watch out for any damages.

Their method comes rather close to our certified milk, which was conceived more than sixty years ago by a practicing physician, Dr. Henry L. Coit, of Newark, New Jersey. In 1893, Coit laid down seventy rules for the production of certified milk and organized the first Medical Milk Commission. Modern methods and skills have influenced Coit's original standards, but his basic plan is still in operation. Certified milk is clean, fresh and very nutritious. Naturally the more nutritious a cow's diet is, the more nutritive values there are in her milk. Nutrition-control for cows producing certified milk begins with the soil and carries through to the actual feeding of the cow. Strict laboratory control standards of cows' rations assure maximum nutritional values and year-round uniform quality, and special precautions protect the nutritional content and flavor of certified milk.

On the other hand, our practice of pasteurization has not won general approval. Apparently there is evidence that this process reduces certain health-giving qualities of milk. It makes the protein of milk greatly inferior to raw protein essential for the body because one of the many enzymes known to science is destroyed and this enzyme is important for assimilation of the minerals in the milk. When they test to make sure that the milk is properly pasteurized, they test for the enzyme phosphatase.

One quality of health which is injured or maybe destroyed by heating, especially if prolonged, is Vitamin C. In pasteurization, the heat is brought to 140 degrees Fahrenheit and kept there for half-an-hour. A further defect of pasteurized milk has been revealed by the work of A. L. Daniels and G. Stearns in an article published in the *American Journal of Biological Chemistry*, Volume XXXVII (1919): "Observing the children who were put on pasteurized milk, and then on raw milk quickly brought to a boiling point and cooled . . . the latter brought much better results in health and weight." They thought that pasteurization leads to the precipitation of the necessary calcium-phosphate salts. They were convinced that prolonged heat limits the health-giving properties of the milk. Although souring also destroys certain qualities of the milk, some scientists still prefer it to pasteurization.

VEGETABLES

Vegetables play a great part in the daily diet of the Hunzakuts. What they grow is similar to our foods, but they eat them mostly raw. Because of the scarcity of fuel they do a limited amount of cooking. There is very little wood available, and no coal or gas.

They grow spinach, lettuce, carrots, peas, turnips, squash, young leaves and various herbs, and they sprout pulses and eat them. It is a popular custom to use herbs in cooking and salads, and herb tea is a great favorite. Potatoes and radishes are eaten frequently.

When they cook their vegetables it is done in a covered vessel so that the light doesn't destroy the nutrients. The method is comparable to our steaming rather than boiling. The fire is kept small, giving the food a chance to simmer in its own juices instead of boiling them away. Very little water is added, and if so the water in which the vegetables are cooked is served with it, or drunk later, but it is never thrown away. Some of the nutritional value of vegetables always remains in the water in which they are cooked. By throwing this water away, phosphorus, calcium, iron, iodine and many other valuable nutrients go down the drain and enrich your garbage pail while your organs suffer for lack of them.

Naturally the Hunza vegetables come straight from the garden.

They simply wash off the dirt and eat them raw for the most part or cook them with the skin on. They never soak their vegetables or scrub the skin from them as we do. The skin contains valuable mineral salts, some of which are lost in soaking, vigorous scrubbing or peeling.

The vegetables have a rich flavor and delicious taste in spite of the fact that there is no seasoning available. But there is no need for it, as the food grown in mineral-rich soil has a natural flavor. In fact the vegetables and fruits in Hunza surpass in looks and flavor any I have ever tasted anywhere else.

Unfortunately, in this country, because we are using chemical sprays (DDT and various other dangerous poisons), we must wash and scrub our vegetables and fruits carefully and even peel them, consequently we lose part of the valuable ingredients in the skin. Then, besides scrubbing vegetables and fruits, we cook our food over high heat and thus destroy more of the valuable ingredients. By the time we consume the food, it is robbed of the necessary nutrients our body requires for good health.

God created man as a healthy individual, and thus man should learn to cherish this and do everything in his power to choose a sensible pattern to retain a healthy and youthful body.

SALADS

Salads are a relevant part of every meal and are served plain, with a dressing of grape vinegar* and an apricot-kernel oil on the side to be used if desired.

A variety of vegetable combinations are cut up for salads, freshly picked from the garden, or the whole vegetable is served.

MEAT

The Hunzas are not vegetarians. However, meat is indeed a rare pleasure! Livestock is not abundant, because animals such as cows, sheep and goats must be fed, and food is scarce, as pasture land is limited. Therefore, meat is scarce, too, and is served only at some special occasions, usually during holidays and weddings.

But when an animal is butchered, the entire edible portion of the carcass is used. Meat is usually prepared in the form of a stew. It is cut up and mixed with vegetables, covered tightly and allowed

* Recipe for grape vinegar on page 109.

to simmer slowly until very tender. Pounded wheat or millet is added to the soup. Rice is served with the stew for variety.

Since chickens have a natural urge to peck at seeds, and since seeds are more valuable than money in Hunza, until recently no chickens were allowed in the state. Now that they have imported a few, eggs have become a great luxury. As there are no dogs in Hunza, the children have also discovered that a chicken, if raised properly, makes a fine family pet. In certain households, the chickens literally "rule the roost."

FRUITS

In Hunza apples, pears, peaches, apricots, black and red cherries and mulberries are grown in large quantities.

Apricots are eaten raw in summer and sun-dried for the winter months. Even the stones of the fresh apricot are cracked open and the kernels also eaten. It is tasty and apparently very nourishing. In fact another food has been discovered in that kernel, mainly a rich oil used by the Hunzakuts in abundance.

We are taught that the diet should consist of proteins, carbohydrates, fats, minerals, vitamins, water and oxygen. However, it is doubtful that the Hunzakuts are aware of these important facts.

The few cows and goats don't produce enough milk to fulfill their daily requirements of fats, so the Hunzakut woman had to search for another source of fat to supplement her family's diet and to make the food more appetizing. By instinct, or natural wisdom, she found it in the most unlikely suspect—the seed of the apricot. And ever since, this knowledge has been passed on from mother to daughter, as it is a complicated method which requires know-how and patience.

Since apricot oil is so essential for their diet, every farmer grows more apricot trees than any of the other fruit trees. It is even said that the maiden's choice of a husband depends on how many apricot trees he owns. A woman cannot own any land if she decides to remain single or when she becomes a widow, but she retains the ownership of the apricot trees.

Inasmuch as there is a trace of prussic acid in the seed and an excess of it could be harmful, one man is assigned to supervise the apricot trees. His job is to taste the fruit of each newly producing tree as well as the seed, and if there is any trace of bitterness the tree is destroyed. The soil rich in minerals bears high-quality fruit, and each tree is covered from bottom to top with an abundance of large-size, luscious-looking fruit.

When the Mir spoke about the soil he said, "It is a gift of God, and it should be treasured as such and worked for."

Scientists have found this apricot oil rich in polyunsaturated fatty acids. One of the greatest benefits of the oil is its remarkable richness in food value. The freedom from circulatory disease, heart attacks and strokes that the Hunzakuts enjoy makes one wonder. There must be a connection between the way they eat and the way they live. Their old men can scale high mountains or work in the fields all day without a trace of fatigue.

Today the apricot is not only the most popular fruit, it is also the most versatile. Its oil is used in cooking, salad dressings, as a food supplement and for medicine, and it is even used as a cosmetic on their skin and hair. Men, women and children use this oil, and it is obvious that it brings excellent results, as most all of them have beautiful skin and lovely hair.

Making the oil is a tedious job, and it is usually left to the women. However, the whole family congregates on the roof of the house to help. First the seeds must be removed from the pits, then pounded into a pulp and rolled into a fine meal with a stone. Then the fine meal is lightly sprinkled with water and heated on a low fire. Finally, as the oil begins to separate from the meal, the pot is removed from the fire and the pulp is kneaded by hand until a generous supply of oil is extracted from the mass. In a final stage the oil is scooped into a jar and allowed to cool. The finished product has a rich, golden-brown color.

Until recently there was no apricot kernel oil available in this country. However, I am glad to learn that a company in California is now manufacturing apricot kernel oil to be used in food.

This particular apricot kernel oil has a delightful almond taste and gives a delicious flavor to salad dressings. It also has an advantage over other oils, because it does not turn rancid readily.

Dried apricots are soaked overnight in rich mineral water and eaten with cooked millet or made into a paste as jam or bread; by adding more water, and then mashing, it is made into juice for drinking. The fruit is very sweet so it serves as a sweetener as well. Apricots have a rich source of organic copper and iron, which might well be the reason for the absence of anemia in the Hunza people.

Hunzakuts seldom cook their fruit. They eat it raw as it comes from the trees. When we were traveling, our drivers would eat a few apricots, crack the seed open with their teeth [indicating a strong dental structure], eat the kernel and be satisfied. Observing their endurance, there was no doubt in my mind that they were nourished well.

It has been established that fresh fruit is an excellent food and good for one's health. This has certainly worked for the Hunza-kuts, for their fruit is pure and fresh and eaten in its unchanged, natural state. Ripened on the tree, it carries the additional quality of a direct relationship between the sun and the fruit. As if by some infallible instinct, the people of Hunza have chosen the richest fruits for cultivation.

Peaches are rich in vitamins and minerals and are prized by the Hunzakuts next to the apricots.

Cherries are an excellent fruit, as the root of the tree penetrates deep into the soil and thus a large supply of minerals and trace elements are found in the fruit. Black cherries and red cherries grow profusely. During my visit the cherries were just ripe and they were served fresh with each meal. They were sweet, juicy and meaty. A few cherries keep one well nourished, as they are rich in iron and are an excellent blood-builder.

The pear, like the apple, had its origin in Asia Minor and Eastern Europe. It has a decided astringent and disinfecting action because of its tannic-acid content. It also contains many mineral salts, including potassium.

The old saying "An apple a day keeps the doctor away" still holds true in Hunza. Apples contain some protein, a trace of fat (oil) and a considerable amount of carbohydrates. They are also an excellent cleaner of teeth. The acid of an apple acts as a potent germicide in the mouth. Also, chewing an apple massages the gums.

Fred D. Miller, D.D., in his book *Open Door to Health*, recommends an apple after each meal.

Grapes are rich in sugar and iron. In Europe many health spas and sanitoriums practice the grape-mono diet (when you eat nothing but grapes) with excellent results. Grapes are low in protein but rich in vitamins and minerals.

WINE

The Hunzas drink freely of their fresh homemade wine, prepared from grapes which are left to ferment for ninety days before using. I found it most delicious, and during my visit with the royal family I enjoyed a glass of wine before the evening meal. It is quite potent, so one glass was sufficient if one wished to remain sober. The Hunza brand is made without sugar, is naturally fermented and, like Hunza fruits and vegetables, is always fresh and alive.

The more orthodox Moslems are teetotalers and disapprove of this habit. But the Hunzas continue to drink their wine.

A DIET WITHOUT POISON

Lacking the facilities for storing fresh fruits and vegetables, the people of Hunza gather them as needed. Their fruit comes straight from the gardens and their vegetables directly from the fields. Ignorant of advanced science and nutrition, they have kept free from disease by using their common sense. Of course, we might say that isolation has been a contributing factor. However, that is not completely so. The Mir has had contact with other countries and could have been influenced by the methods of other peoples. But he was not, and they have continued using the primitive methods established centuries ago.

The Rani told me of the time insects invaded an area of Pakistan and Hunza was visited by an official of the Pakistani government to arrange for the spraying of their gardens. She forbade it. She simply had ashes put in the water and the insects did not return. That summer the crop was not as abundant but it wasn't contaminated by poisonous sprays.

Some months later the Rani visited relatives in Nagir. Upon sitting down to a royal dinner, she learned that the plants of Nagir had been sprayed by pesticides. She was horrified and refused to eat at all during her stay. The idea of eating such poison was unthinkable to her.

The Hunzakuts have not even followed the "civilized" practices of their neighbors. They have remained faithful to their customs and thereby preserved the purity of their valley.

ON THE BENEFITS OF RAW FOODS

"Of all arts, the art of healing is the most distinguished," said Hippocrates, the father of medicine. His philosophy called for a physician to possess not only knowledge and experience but also a discerning personality. He also stated, "The philosophy-loving physician is God-resembling."

Hippocrates believed in fasting, plenty of sleep, exercises and morning walks. Coarse whole-grain bread, fruits and raw vegetables were recommended to his patients. He told them, "Your food should be your medicine. . . ."

How similar to the Hunzas pattern of eating and living!

If people were taught to eat more raw fruits and vegetables, malnutrition and dietary deficiencies would decrease greatly. The Hunza diet consists mostly of raw fruits and vegetables, plus an abundance of whole grains. What we consider lack of comfort has kept the Hunzas healthy and happy.

In a diet of raw food, the enzymes, which cannot stand high temperatures, are kept intact, and this is one of the main reasons raw foods are superior to cooked foods. On the other hand, when foods are cooked, the proteins become coagulated, making them less digestible. Some of the important amino acids of the protein, such as cystine and cysteine, are changed by the heat and water to such an extent that they no longer have the same nutritional value.

The idea of eating raw foods may be unappealing to some people, but as one learns the benefits to be derived from foods in their natural state, it becomes easier to accept them. Eventually they are preferred and become a pleasant habit. The housewife can learn to prepare tasty dishes of raw vegetables and fruits in a variety of salads. Healthful foods should look appetizing and should be tasty. Your family will learn to enjoy such meals if a little effort and interest is expended in their preparation.

An experiment made by the State Institute of Food Research in Denmark during World War II brought some startling facts to light. The Danes imported grain from the United States for human as well as domestic-animal consumption. During the blockade no new grain could be brought in. The Danes faced the dilemma of feeding whatever grain they had to their animals and virtually starving themselves, or starving most of the animals and keeping the grain for themselves. Of course, they chose the latter. After their supply of meat was exhausted they subsisted largely on whole grains in the form of cereals and bread, and plenty of green and root vegetables, dairy products and fruit. The healthful results of this enforced limited diet was remarkable. It matched almost exactly the Hunza diet—whole-grain meals, vegetables, fruit, dairy products and very little meat.

10.

Recipes from the Rooftop of the World

The following recipes were collected during my stay in Hunza. Most of them are original Hunza dishes, others have been collected by the Rani from around the world. Some of the original ingredients have been changed to ingredients readily available in this country.

✑§ APPETIZERS ଡ଼

ORANGE, CHERRY AND CANTALOUPE SUPREME

1½ cups deep red cherries
3 cups cantaloupe balls or cubes
½ cup lemon juice

½ cup orange juice
3 tablespoons raw sugar or honey

Wash and pit the cherries. Arrange the melon balls or cubes in cocktail glasses with cherries, diced orange pulp, and sugar. Add 2 tablespoons of orange and lemon juice, mixed, to each portion. Serves 12.

FRUIT SUPREME

½ cup pineapple, diced
½ cup orange, diced
½ cup grapefruit, diced
½ cup seedless raisins

⅓ cup grape juice
1 cup cold water (bottled)
yogurt or sour cream topping

Combine the fruits; then add the grape juice diluted with the water. Let stand for twenty minutes. Remove the fruit and put into chilled cocktail glasses. Add grape juice and top with yogurt or sour cream. Serves 4.

FRUIT HORS D'OEUVRES PLATE

Arrange groups of the following on a serving plate or platter and allow each person to help himself. Use a base of shredded lettuce. Prepare according to the number to be served and serve very cold soon after making:

Orange sections Remove all membrane and if desired roll in toasted coconut. The translucence of the fruit is attractive without coconut, however.

Orange slices Cut with scissors at each place where sections join, spreading apart flowerlike. Center with mayonnaise and a slice of stuffed olive.

Melon balls Roll in fine coconut.

Berries or apricot halves Roll in chopped mint.

Pineapple sections Roll in chopped nuts.

Banana sections Marinate in lemon juice to prevent darkening. Decorate with star of sour cream or yogurt.

Dates and prunes Remove stones; then stuff with cream cheese and ground nuts moistened with lemon juice. (Cottage cheese may be used.)

Lemon baskets Make the baskets from lemon rind and fill with almonds.

Variations For the fruits given, other fruits may be substituted in season, such as pears, peaches and berries.

VARIOUS FRUIT COMBINATIONS

Mix directly in each of four serving glasses (for larger portions increase amount accordingly) any of the following combinations:

⅓ cup cantaloupe cubes or balls; ⅓ cup fresh red raspberries; ¼ cup fresh orange juice.

⅓ cup black raspberries; ⅓ cup diced yellow peaches; ⅓ cup unsweetened pineapple juice.

⅓ cup fresh apricot wedges; ⅓ cup purple grape halves or seeded black cherries. Sweeten to taste with honey.

Diced papaya may be added to any of above combinations if available.

MUSHROOM AND PARSLEY CANAPE

Cook 6 large mushrooms* in butter until tender. Allow to cool, then slice and place on whole-wheat toast shapes. Sprinkle with minced parsley and season with a few drops of lemon juice. Makes 6 canapés.

TOMATO AND EGG CANAPES

8 rounds whole-wheat bread	hard-cooked eggs, sliced
2 tablespoons mayonnaise	natural mineral salt
sliced tomatoes	4 stuffed green olives, sliced

Toast rounds of bread on one side and spread the untoasted side with mayonnaise. Add thin slices of tomato, then slices of hard-cooked egg. Sprinkle very lightly with vegetable salt and garnish with a slice or two of stuffed olives. Makes 8 canapés.

COLD SHRIMP HORS D'OEUVRES

8 fresh, cooked, cleaned shrimp	curry powder
8 rounds whole-wheat bread	parsley
¼ cup mayonnaise	8 drops Worcestershire sauce

* Raw mushrooms can be used if desired.

Place shrimp on round of whole-wheat bread cut same size. Top each shrimp with mayonnaise, season with a drop of Worcestershire sauce and a dash of curry powder. Garnish with sprig of parsley. Makes 8 hors d'oeuvres.

AVOCADO COCKTAIL

Place avocado balls in cocktail glasses. Cover with chilled dressing made by blending 1 part lemon juice, 2 parts orange juice and dash of salt.

AVOCADO PASTE

2 avocados, natural mineral salt to taste; juice of ½ lemon or more if desired; 2 tablespoons apricot-kernel oil; ½ cup yogurt. Blend well. This is excellent for a dip or on sandwiches.

৵ SOUPS ৶

VEGETABLE BROTH

Chop 3 cups of various vegetables—carrots, turnips, celery, broccoli, leek, parsnips, cabbage, parsley, etc. Blend in blender with 4 cups of water and simmer covered for a few minutes over low heat. Season to taste with vegetable salt, add 1 tablespoon butter and serve unstrained. Makes 3 cups.

VEGETABLE CHOWDER

1 cup shredded lettuce	4 tablespoons apricot-kernel oil
1 cup shredded celery	2 cups boiling water
1 medium-sized onion	vegetable salt
2 medium-sized carrots, cut	½ cup millet (precooked)

Chop vegetables, heat oil in saucepan, add vegetables and simmer for about five minutes. Add water and simmer over low heat for another five minutes. Stir in cooked millet, season to taste and serve. Makes 3 cups.

POTATO SOUP

2 medium-sliced potatoes
2 medium-sized onions
5 carrots

½ teaspoon vegetable salt; paprika
2 tablespoons butter
milk or stock (vegetable or chicken)

Peel and slice potatoes, chop onions and carrots. Cook vegetables in small amount of stock until tender, put through a ricer or in liquefier. Beat in butter and thin soup to desired consistency with milk or additional stock, sprinkle with salt, paprika and garnish with chopped parsley before serving. Makes 4 cups.

CREAM OF SPINACH

2 pounds spinach
2 tablespoons apricot-kernel oil
vegetable salt; paprika

4 cups water
4 teaspoons vege-broth
1 tablespoon grated onion

Wash spinach well. While moist place in covered saucepan and cook for six minutes. Put through a strainer. Preheat oil in skillet and sauté grated onions for five minutes over low heat. Stir in gradually 4 cups of vege-broth (1 teaspoon vege-soup powder to 1 cup boiling water), simmer slowly for five minutes. Season with salt and paprika, add spinach and heat well. Serve with wheat croutons. Makes 5 cups.

CREAM OF TOMATO

2 cups tomatoes
½ cup chopped celery
¼ cup chopped onion
2 teaspoons honey

4 cups raw milk
4 tablespoons butter
vegetable salt; paprika

Simmer vegetables in small amount water for fifteen minutes, add milk slowly to prevent curdling. Season and simmer over low heat for another ten minutes. Blend in butter and honey just before serving and serve with brown rice cooked separately. Makes 6 cups.

BORSCH

2 cups beets	1 cucumber
1 cup carrots	1 cup finely shredded cabbage
1 cup onions	sour cream or yogurt
1 teaspoon vegetable salt	2 teaspoons honey (more if desired)
1 tablespoon butter	

Peel and chop fine beets, carrots and onions, cover with water and boil gently over low heat, covered, for about twenty minutes. Add 2 cups of water, blend in butter, salt, honey, lemon and cabbage. Simmer for another ten minutes or until vegetables are tender. Serve in bowls, adding a tablespoon of sour cream or yogurt in each, and garnish with chopped parsley if desired. Makes 6 cups.

MILLET SOUP

1 small head cabbage	¾ cup celery and parsley mixed
1 quart vegetable or meat stock	½ teaspoon seasoning
1 cup millet meal or whole millet	1 tablespoon apricot-kernel oil if desired
½ cup chopped onion	

Cook onion and celery with a little water until tender. Wet millet meal until all is damp. If whole millet is used cook for about fifteen minutes. Add liquid and millet to the onion, parsley and celery mixture and cook slowly until cabbage is tender. Stir in parsley and seasonings and salt to taste just before serving. Makes 6 soup plates.

Note: Leftover cooked vegetables may be used in place of the cabbage.

✎§ CHAPATTI §✎

In Hunza, chapattis are eaten with every meal instead of bread. They are made out of whole-wheat grains, stoneground daily.

CHAPATTI (basic recipe)

2 cups whole-wheat flour	¾ to 1 cup water
½ teaspoon salt	

Blend flour and salt together. Stir just enough water to make a very stiff dough. Knead dough on a lightly floured surface until smooth and elastic. Cover with a wet cloth; set aside for thirty minutes.

Break the dough off, form into 1-inch balls, and roll out into very thin rounds, about 8 inches in diameter.

Bake on both sides on a lightly greased griddle over low heat. Delicious rolled paper thin and served with thick sour cream. Makes 20 chapattis.

PRATHAS CHAPATTI

2 cups whole-wheat flour (freshly stoneground)	¼ pound butter
½ cup water	½ teaspoon sea salt

Mix butter with flour then blend water in a little at a time. Roll dough ½ inch thick and bake on preheated griddle greased with butter. Makes 8 chapattis.

READY-MIX CHAPATTI (basic recipe)

1 egg well beaten	3 tablespoons ready-mix*
2 tablespoons water	

Blend well and, with a spoon, dish out on a preheated skillet greased with apricot-kernel oil small, thin pancakes about 5 inches in diameter. Then cover with a lid for a few minutes over very low fire. Turn over and brown it on the other side for a few minutes. Serve with honey or slices of cheese. Makes approximately 3 thin chapatti pancakes.

CHEESE CHAPATTI

½ cup whole-wheat flour	3¼ cups buttermilk
1½ cups buckwheat flour	2 eggs
½ teaspoon baking powder	2 tablespoons butter or apricot-kernel oil
½ teaspoon vegetable salt	

Sift flour, salt and baking powder together. Add buttermilk and oil. Beat egg yolks and add. Beat batter until smooth and elastic.

* The reader may write the author for information on obtaining Ready-Mix Chapatti, which will be available in stores.

Then add the stiffly beaten egg whites. Bake chapattis on a medium-hot griddle following customary rules. Makes 8 large chapattis.

FILLING

coriander greens   2 cups cottage cheese

Blend cottage cheese with buttermilk until smooth. Add vegetable salt to taste and chopped coriander greens. Lay out 1 chapatti and spread cheese all over, cover with another and repeat until all are used. Let stand for two hours then cut like a cake and serve.

✎§ VEGETABLES §✎

SPINACH CURRY*

Wash well and drain 2 pounds of fresh spinach. Let stand for a while. Shortly before serving blend in a liquefier, including the juice, then warm the spinach in a double boiler, adding about 1 teaspoon of natural mineral salt to taste, ½ teaspoon Spike,** 2 teaspoons curry powder and cook slowly for about five minutes or until heated through thoroughly. Add 2 tablespoons of apricot-kernel oil and ¼ pound ground almonds. Mix and serve hot. Serves 6.

Omit the curry and after removing from the heat, stir slowly one cup of yogurt or sour cream and then sprinkle with fresh chopped parsley. Serves 6.

HUNZA SPINACH IN CHAPATTIS

Prepare creamed spinach according to basic recipe, adding chopped mushrooms sautéed in apricot-kernel oil. Blend. Make thin chapattis according to recipe ready-mix chapatti. Place a large tablespoon of spinach mixture on each chapatti, roll them and serve with yogurt or sour cream.

* Same spinach recipe can be used for creamed spinach.
** Dr. Gaylord Hauser's vegetable salt with herbs.

FRUITED CREAMED SPINACH

Using same method as for creamed spinach, ½ cup of pineapple juice and juice of ½ lemon. Heat in double boiler. Before serving stir 2 tablespoons of apricot-kernel oil, sprinkle with fresh parsley and chopped almonds.

FRESH GREEN PEAS (fresh only)

Cook peas over low heat in well-covered pan. Chop fine green scallions and add to the peas during cooking. When ready, season to taste with mineral salt and Spike, and add a tablespoon of apricot-kernel oil. Before serving, sprinkle with chopped parsley.

BOILED ONIONS

Take 2 pounds of white onions. Boil slowly over low heat until done. (It is preferable to use waterless, stainless-steel dishes for cooking vegetables.) Mash onions in liquidizer, add a cup of buttermilk, mineral salt and mint leaves to taste. Mix well and then heat through just before serving. Serves 6.

EGGPLANT

Cut a medium-sized eggplant crosswise into slices ½ inch thick. Sauté the eggplant in apricot-kernel oil over low heat. Turn over to brown on both sides. Turn off the heat. Sprinkle with ½ cup grated cheese, or place small slices of cheese on each eggplant, cover with lid until cheese melts. Serves 3.

EGGPLANT CASSEROLE

2 medium-sized eggplants	6 cups milk
4 cups bread crumbs (whole wheat)	6 eggs
2 teaspoons mineral salt	1 teaspoon rosemary
other herbs can be used	

Peel and cube eggplants. Cook in salted water five minutes. Beat eggs and add milk, and pour over bread crumbs. Add to bread and egg all remaining ingredients. Pour into an oiled baking dish, place dish in pan of hot water, and bake in 350° oven for forty-five minutes or until set. Serves 10.

MILLET CASSEROLE

1 cup hulled millet
½ cup diced carrots
½ cup diced celery
1 tablespoon chopped pimento

2 tablespoons safflower oil
1 teaspoon vegetable salt
1 teaspoon salad herbs

Heat oil in heavy skillet, stir in millet and brown slightly. Add chopped vegetables, salt and stir for three minutes. Put millet into a covered saucepan, adding enough water to cover about 1 inch above the millet. Cook over low heat for fifteen minutes. Then continue cooking in a double boiler until tender. Serves 6.

QUICK WILD RICE

½ cup wild rice
½ cup boiling water

½ tablespoon vegetable salt
1 tablespoon butter or safflower oil

Add rice to boiling, salted water. Cover and cook over slow heat without stirring for twenty minutes. Remove cover, dot oil or butter over top and let stand few minutes in warm place to dry out. Serve with fowl or lamb stew. Serves 4.

HUNZA RICE WITH ALMONDS OR NUTS

2 pounds brown rice
butter or apricot-kernel oil
¼ pound almonds or nuts

¼ pound raisins
4 large onions
salt to taste

Cook rice in the usual manner. Brown onions in a skillet in apricot-kernel oil. Sprinkle over rice, then add chopped almonds or nuts and raisins. Serves 10.

GREEN RICE

3 cups cooked brown rice
2 cups grated cheese
2 tablespoons minced onion
1 cup chopped parsley

3 cups milk or half-and-half
½ cup mayonnaise
3 eggs beaten
2 teaspoons mineral salt

Cook and drain rice beforehand. Chop parsley very fine and mix with rice, onion, grated cheese and salt. Add mayonnaise. Last, add beaten eggs and milk and blend well. Pour into oiled baking dish. Set in pan of hot water and bake at 375° until set. Serves 4.

NAI CHORU (saffron rice)

¼ cup safflower oil
½ cup chopped onion
1 cup uncooked brown rice
½ teaspoon vegetable salt
⅛ teaspoon ground cloves

few grains ground saffron
1½ cups water
⅓ cup toasted slivered almonds
⅓ cup dark seedless raisins

Heat cooking oil in heavy skillet. Add onion and cook over low heat until soft, stirring occasionally. Add rice and brown lightly, stirring frequently. Add water and salt, cloves and saffron. Mix well. Cover and cook over low heat fifteen to twenty minutes or until all water is absorbed and rice is tender. Lightly mix in almonds and raisins. This dish is especially good served with lamb curries. Serves 6.

VEGETABLE CURRY

2 pounds assorted raw vegetables
¼ cup apricot-kernel oil or sesame
3 tablespoons grated coconut
1½ tablespoons curry powder

1 teaspoon vegetable mineral salt
3 tomatoes, peeled and diced
1½ cups water or meat broth

Prepare vegetables and set aside. Vegetable suggestions: kohlrabi, turnips or potatoes, diced; carrots, sliced; celery, diced; cabbage, cut up. Warm up oil in large, heavy skillet. Add coconut and garlic and cook until onion is soft, stirring occasionally. Blend in vegetables and water. Cover and bring to boiling, over low heat, stirring occasionally. Cook until vegetables are tender. Serves 4 to 6.

BROCCOLI

2 bunches fresh broccoli
1 teaspoon vegetable salt
¼ cup almonds, slivered
juice of ½ lemon

1 tablespoon safflower oil
    or apricot-kernel oil
½ cup yogurt

Cut broccoli into small pieces. Moisten and then sauté, covered, over heat for about ten minutes or until tender. Add vegetable salt. Drain, reserving liquid for soup (never throw away any of your vegetable liquids). Sprinkle with lemon juice, oil. Mix lightly, then top with yogurt and sprinkle with almonds. Serve at once. Serves 6.

BANANA SQUASH

Using 1 loose cup shredded banana squash per serving, prepare squash by cutting in small pieces, heat slightly and blend with a little water just to keep it moist. Add mineral salt to taste, 1 teaspoon apricot-kernel oil and ½ teaspoon honey. Heat to 115° and serve.

STUFFED CELERY

1 cup tahini (sesame-seed butter)
5½ ounces lemon juice
¾ cup chopped green pepper
3 tablespoons honey

1 cup minced parsley
1 cup chopped ripe olives
2 teaspoons ground sage
2 teaspoons mineral salt

Delicious spread on celery or apple slices.

CAULIFLOWER

1 head cauliflower, finely grated
2 tablespoons minced parsley

3 tablespoons apricot-kernel oil
mineral salt to taste

Heat to 115° and serve. Makes 6 portions.

WHOLE BUCKWHEAT GROATS

1 cup whole buckwheat groats
2 cups water
1 egg

1 teaspoon Spike
2 tablespoons safflower oil

Heat oil in heavy skillet, stir in the buckwheat groats mixed with the beaten whole egg. Add the salt and brown slightly, keeping it stirred with a spoon. Finally, add the water, bring to a boil, then reduce heat, cover tightly and let simmer until all liquid is absorbed. It should not be mushy. Every grain should be separate. Serves 6.

OATMEAL CEREAL (birchermuesl)

2 tablespoons raw oatmeal
water
1 apple, grated

1 tablespoon honey
juice of ½ lemon
½ cup yogurt*

Soak raw oatmeal in water overnight. Stir well next morning and add the grated apple, honey and lemon juice. Blend in the yogurt and serve at once. Serves 2.

MILLET HULLED

½ cup hulled millet**
1 cup water (bottled)
1 cup milk

1 tablespoon honey
½ teaspoon Spike (vegetable salt)
dried apricots, soaked overnight

Heat water and milk in top of double boiler. Add millet and steam over boiling water for thirty minutes or until millet is tender. Serve hot. Add dried apricots and honey. Serves 4.

BEAUTY SALAD

1 head of lettuce, cut up
4 Jerusalem artichokes
2 tomatoes
1 cup of alfalfa sprouts

1 avocado
3 stalks diced celery
1 green pepper, shredded
3 carrots, shredded

* Milk or half-and-half may be used instead of yogurt. The Hunzas use yogurt most of the time, considering it a very nourishing food.
** Millet is very rich in protein and the Hunza people use it in large quantities as a cereal.

Mix the ingredients well in a salad bowl. Blend salad dressing, then top with slices of tomatoes, avocado and sprinkle with alfalfa sprouts. Serves 6.

DRESSING

Mix 2 tablespoons apricot-kernel oil, 1 tablespoon apple-cider vinegar, 1 teaspoon honey, 1 teaspoon natural-mineral salt, ½ teaspoon Spike and juice of a whole lemon. Shake well and pour over vegetables.

❧ MEAT ☙

LEG OF LAMB (basic recipe*)

1 leg of lamb	½ cup of red wine (Hunzas use
2 medium onions	grape wine, homemade)
1 orange	vegetable salt
3 carrots	garlic powder
5 small potatoes (young)	savory
	herbs

Cut off all fat, then place leg of lamb under the hot-water faucet and let hot water run over it for about five minutes. Pierce a few points with a sharp knife to allow it to absorb as much water as possible. Make a dry mixture of the seasonings and rub well into the meat. Insert a few slivers of garlic into the surface of the meat. Place in shallow baking pan or roaster with a lid. Pour 1 cup of cold water over the meat and place in preheated 350° oven for about thirty minutes. Reduce the temperature to 300° and roast twenty minutes per pound. Cut onions into quarters and place in pan with carrots and potatoes. Baste meat frequently with drippings, adding more cold water when necessary, pouring over the roast. Half an hour before meat is done, place slivers of orange on top of meat and baste with wine.

*Same recipe can be used for fowl. Pineapple, peaches or apricots can be used instead of oranges. But always wash meat or fowl with hot water (same method as above) to get enough moisture into the meat before placing it in the oven.

MINCED LAMB CURRY IN CHAPATTIS

2 pounds lamb, minced (cooked)
1 cup water or meat broth
1 teaspoon curry powder

1 teaspoon vegetable salt, or to
    taste and onion salt (optional)

Mix meat well with seasonings and moisten meat with water or broth. Prepare 2 large chapattis, uncooked (see basic recipe for chapattis), place meat in between, pressing edges together, and place in oiled pan or skillet and cook on slow fire until chapattis are done, or bake in a 300° oven. Serves 6. (Can be served with yogurt and sprinkled with chopped parsley.)

HUNZA MUTTON-BALL CURRY

2 pounds lamb, minced
1 cup water
2 teaspoons seasonings (vegetable
    salt, pepper, curry powder)

2 onions, chopped fine
2 tablespoons safflower oil
    or any other oil
water

Prepare mutton balls by combining minced meat with 1 cup of water and seasonings. Sauté onions in safflower oil until tender and golden, do not brown. Add 1 quart of water, bring to a boil, then add the meat balls and cook over low heat for about twenty minutes. Remove meat balls and allow soup to boil down to about 2 cups. Again add meat balls and allow to simmer until hot. Serves 6. (Chopped mushrooms sautéed and blended with sour cream may be added for flavor.)

HUNZA MEAT STEW

2 pounds lamb shoulder
1 quart water
1 tablespoon natural-mineral salt
3 small carrots, sliced
2 stalks celery, diced
parsley, bay leaf and sprig-dried
    thyme tied together in a bundle

1 tablespoon lemon juice
10 small onions peeled (white)
    (optional)
¼ pound mushrooms, sliced
2 tablespoons apricot-kernel oil
1 cup of sour cream

Cut lamb into small pieces, cover with water and bring to a boil. Skim off all excess fat. Add bundle of herbs and simmer until meat is almost tender. Add onions, salt, carrots and celery and continue simmering for about thirty minutes. Sauté the mushrooms in oil in separate pan for about five minutes over low heat. Add to stew. Beat the sour cream with lemon juice and pour in some of the hot gravy, mixing briskly. Add to the stew and cook a few minutes below boiling point. Do not allow mixture to boil. Sprinkle with chopped parsley. Serves 6.

INDIAN LAMB STEW

2 pounds boneless lamb,
    cut in 1- to 1½-inch pieces
2 tablespoons apricot-kernel oil
2 teaspoons natural mineral salt
½ teaspoon Spike
2 cups water

1 package frozen or fresh green peas
    (10 ounces)
2 teaspoons curry powder
1 small clove of garlic, minced
½ cup chopped onion
1 tablespoon lemon juice

Brown lamb in oil, add salt, curry powder, garlic, onion and water. Cover kettle tightly and simmer slowly for 1½ hours or until lamb is tender. Add peas and cook until peas are done. Stir in lemon juice. Serves 6.

INDIAN LAMB CURRY

¼ cup apricot-kernel oil
1 pound boneless lamb shoulder
    cut in 1-inch cubes
½ cup chopped onion
1 clove garlic, minced

3 tablespoons packaged grated
    coconut
1 tablespoon curry powder
1 chili pepper, finely chopped
2 cups beef broth

Heat 2 tablespoons oil in large, heavy skillet. Lightly coat lamb pieces with whole-wheat flour. Add meat to skillet and brown evenly over medium heat. Remove meat from skillet with a slotted spoon and set aside.

Add remaining oil, onion, garlic and coconut to skillet; cook until onion is soft, stirring occasionally. Stir in curry powder, chili pepper, broth and browned meat. Cover and simmer for about one hour, stirring occasionally. Serve with saffron rice and apple chutney. Serves 4.

MEAT LOAF SUPREME

1½ pounds ground beef
1 cup wheat germ
2 eggs, slightly beaten
½ cup water
1 small can tomato sauce

1 teaspoon natural mineral salt
½ teaspoon Spike
2 teaspoons sesame oil
½ teaspoon sage

Mix all ingredients thoroughly. Bake in loaf pan in 350° oven for one hour or until done. Serves 6 or 8.

MEAT — MONTO

2 pounds minced meat (beef or lamb)
1 pound finely chopped onions
natural-mineral salt to taste

various spices can be added
2 tablespoons apricot-kernel oil

Mix well, blending a little bit of water to make the meat soft. Use basic recipe for chapatti (page 86). Roll small pieces the size of a saucer. Put about 2 teaspoons of meat mixture in the center, fold dough over and close tightly with fingers. Place in a steamer until tender. Serve with apricot-kernel oil, butter or sour cream. Serves 6.

SWINGER

(The famous recipe served at the Sunset Strip "Aware Inn" in Los Angeles.)

12 ounces ground sirloin tip
1 egg yolk

1 heaping tablespoon of chopped onions, green peppers, tomatoes, raw Tillamook cheese, olives

Mix well and make into a patty . . . . . Broil . . . . . 1 Serving.

❧ EGGS ❧

FLUFFY OMELET

1 egg
1 tablespoon water
2 tablespoons sour cream or yogurt

½ teaspoon mineral salt
1 tablespoon apricot-kernel oil

Beat the egg yolk well, add water and salt, continuing to beat. Then add yogurt and blend well. Fold in the stiffly beaten egg white. Heat the skillet, add oil, then omelet, cover with a lid and cook slowly over low heat. With a fork or pancake-turner, lift the edges and tilt the skillet to permit the uncooked butter to run to the bottom. When the top is set, fold the omelet in the middle with a spatula, turn off the heat. Top it with a few slices of cheese. Let it melt under the lid and serve it hot. Serves 1.

Another suggestion: Blend half of a 3-ounce package of cream cheese with 2 tablespoons of sour cream or yogurt, mix well and add chopped parsley. Before folding the omelet, spread cream cheese on one side and then fold over. Keep it under the lid for a few minutes. Serve hot.

HUNZA SPINACH EGGS

Fill a buttered baking dish with creamed spinach. Press hollows in the spinach with a large spoon. Break one egg into each hollow. Season to taste with natural-mineral salt or Spike. Place dish in pan of hot water and bake in preheated 325° oven for about ten minutes or until eggs are firm. Sprinkle with chopped parsley. Serves 4.

❧ DESSERTS ❧

APRICOT UP-SIDE-DOWN CAKE

3 tablespoons butter
1 cup brown sugar
1 pound apricots
4 eggs

1 cup stoneground whole-wheat flour
1 teaspoon baking powder
¼ teaspoon salt

Melt butter and add the brown sugar (½ cup). Stir until well blended with the butter. Arrange half of the apricots round-side-down in baking dish and pour the melted butter and sugar mixture around them. Beat 2 whole eggs and 2 yolks. Add the remaining sugar, flour, baking powder and salt and blend well. Fold in the stiffly beaten 2 egg whites. Pour the batter over the apricots and sugar mixture. Bake in a moderate oven, 350° for fifty minutes or until cake is done. Cool slightly and invert the pan on a large plate so that the apricots will be on top. Serve with whipped cream or yogurt whipped with a fork or sour cream. Serves 6.

CREAM CHEESE WHIP*

3-ounce package of cream cheese
3 tablespoon certified raw milk or yogurt

2 tablespoons honey

Blend the cream cheese and yogurt, add the honey and beat until light and fluffy. Serves 6 to 8.

FRUIT TART (basic recipe)

1 cup sour cream
1 cake yeast (fresh)
1 teaspoon brown sugar

2 cups whole-wheat flour
¼ pound sweet butter
pinch sea salt

Mix yeast with sugar to dissolve it into a paste, blend into sour cream and let rise in a warm place for approximately one hour. Mix flour with salt and butter until all the butter is blended smoothly. Combine sour cream-yeast mixture with flour mixture and knead until dough leaves the sides of the bowl. Toss dough in pan for about five minutes. If dough is too soft, add a little flour until it is easily handled. Divide into 4 parts and roll to pie-crust thickness. Bake in oven at 300° until slightly brown. Makes 4 pie crusts.

FILLING

One pound of fresh peaches or any other fruit in season, cut in half, place on crust (baked). Blend well with a fork, 1 cup of yogurt and 1 tablespoon of honey and serve over the fruit.

* Can be used on fresh fruit.

CHEESE TART

1 pint large curd cottage cheese	3 tablespoons honey
2 eggs	1 lemon rind, grated
10 cashew nuts and 10 almonds, chopped	⅛ teaspoon salt

Butter a pie plate, roll out thin the basic tart recipe and bake at 300° for about fifteen minutes or until brown and done.

Mix cottage cheese with beaten egg yolks in a mixing bowl until it is smooth, add honey, vanilla, nuts and lemon rind. Fold in stiffly beaten egg whites. Spoon into baked tart crust and bake in slow oven until cheese firms. Be careful not to overcook. Serves 6.

YOGURT PIE

1 cup thick yogurt	pinch of salt
½ pound cream cheese	½ cup raisins
1 tablespoon honey	¼ cup nuts, chopped fine
grated rind from 1 lemon	½ cup apricots, cut fine (fresh in season,
juice of ½ lemon	dry or frozen out of season)

Whip the filling until smooth. Pour into a pastry shell and place in refrigerator until served. Serves 3.

(To make without a pastry shell, line bottom of pastry dish with wheat-germ flakes.)

FLAKY PIE CRUST

1 cup whole-wheat pastry flour	1 cup wheat germ
1 teaspoon salt	¼ pound sweet butter

Sift flour and salt together into mixing bowl. Add wheat germ. Mix butter with flour until well blended. Sprinkle 4 tablespoons of icewater over mixture, blending until dough leaves sides of bowl completely dry. Place dough between sheets of wax paper, roll out quite thin. Remove wax paper and fit dough into pie plate, easing off the waxed paper. Fill with favorable fruits and cover with top crust rolled out as above. Make a few slits in top crust and bake for ten minutes at 425°. (Makes 2 crusts.)

CREAMY PEAR PIE

5 fresh Bosc or Anjou pears
¾ cup raw sugar
3 tablespoons pastry flour
¼ cup table cream

¼ teaspoon ginger
½ teaspoon nutmeg
pastry for 1 crust, 9-inch pie

Prepare pastry and line pie plate. Pare, core and thinly slice 2 pears into unbaked shell. Halve, pare and core remaining pears. Place halves, cut side down, in circle with stem ends toward center on top of sliced pears. Combine sugar, flour, cream, ginger and nutmeg. Pour over pears. Bake at 425°, forty to forty-five minutes. Makes one 9-inch pie.

CHEESE PIE

pastry for one crust
1 pint cottage cheese
¼ cup milk
¼ cup yogurt or sour cream

1 teaspoon vanilla
4 eggs
¼ cup honey or to taste

Line a pie pan with the pastry. Mix the cheese thoroughly with honey, milk and yogurt until smooth. Blend in slightly beaten egg yolks and then the stiffly beaten egg whites. Pour into the pastry shell, which has been baking in a 300° oven (about ten minutes). Remove pastry from oven and pour in the filling while pastry is hot. Return to oven reduced to 250° and continue baking for ten minutes. Serves 6.

HIGH-PROTEIN PUDDING

1 package gelatin
⅓ cup of cold water
1⅔ cups of hot milk
8 heaping teaspoons of carob
   powder

6 heaping teaspoons of protein
   powder
2 tablespoons of seedless raisins
2 tablespoons chopped walnuts

Sprinkle gelatin on cold water and let it stand. Warm milk gradually over low heat. Add half of the warm milk to gelatin, the other half add to the rest of the ingredients and then, blending well, add nuts and raisins and mix with gelatin. Chill. Serves 4.

APRICOT YOGURT WHIP

1 tablespoon carob powder
1 tablespoon protein powder
1 teaspoon honey

1 tablespoon apricot concentrate
3 tablespoons yogurt

Blend well. Serves 1. (Can be used as topping over fruit.)

WHEAT-GERM CHOCOLATE CAKE

6 eggs
6 teaspoons wheat-germ flour
6 teaspoons carob powder
lemon

1 cup brown sugar
3 teaspoons black coffee
1 cup grated walnuts

Separate egg yolks and mix until smooth with sugar. Grate in lemon rind, squeeze lemon and add juice. Add carob and wheat germ and blend well. Fold in the very stiffly beaten egg whites and mix slowly until it is fluffy and all one color. Pour into cake pan with removable bottom and bake in a 300° oven for ten to fifteen minutes or until consistency is dry when tested with a fork. Cool and ice with following icing.

ICING

½ pound sweet butter
6 teaspoons coffee (liquid)
rind of one lemon

honey to taste (approximately ¼ cup)
1 bar of carob or carob powder
1 egg

Allow butter to stand at room temperature until soft. Cream with a spoon or in an electric mixing bowl until it is soft and fluffy. Add honey and lemon rind and continue to stir until well blended. Then add coffee by the teaspoonful so as not to separate the butter. Melt the chocolate over low heat and stir in raw egg and mix until smooth. Add to the butter and continue to beat until everything takes on one color and is smooth and fluffy. Cover the cake and keep refrigerated. Serves 8 or 10.

🍃 LONGEVITY FROM A LIQUEFIER 🦢

ALMOND MILK

1 tablespoon almond meal
    or ground almonds

1 cup water, bottled
honey to taste

Blend well. Serves 1.

COCONUT MILK

1 cup coconut, grated
honey to taste

2 cups hot water (bottled)

Blend well. Serves 2.

ORANGE BLEND (excellent for breakfast)

2 oranges, thinly peeled, leaving
    white membrane on (cut up in
    blender, including seeds)
½ cup fresh pineapple, diced

2 tablespoons sunflower seed meal
    or almond meal (ground nuts)
honey to taste

Blend just long enough to mix thoroughly. This mixture is quite
thick and can be eaten with a spoon. Serves 3.

APRICOT COMPOTE

Simmer 1 cup of water and ½ cup of honey over low heat until
well blended. Pour hot syrup over halved fresh apricots. Keep in
cool place until ready to serve. (Other fruits may be substituted
for the apricots.)

ORANGE SHERBET

24 ounces orange juice
6 ounces honey
2½ cups papaya cut into small cubes

½ teaspoon sea salt
3 ounces lemon juice

Blend the ingredients in a blender until smooth and then freeze. Serves 4.

APRICOT WHIP

1 package dried apricots, washed and soaked overnight in bottled water. Sweeten to taste with honey. Blend in liquefier to smooth consistency. Add 1 cup of cold yogurt whipped with a fork before serving. Serves 4.

PRUNE-APRICOT WHIP

1 cup soaked dried apricots   **1 cup soaked dried prunes**

Soak fruit overnight using enough bottled water to cover fruit. At least one cup of liquid from the soaked fruit and the fruit itself should be placed in a blender and blended until smooth, adding water if necessary to keep moisture moving in blender and to keep motor from stalling. Top with almond milk. Serves 3.

PINEAPPLE WHIP

1 fresh pineapple   **3 tablespoons honey**
1 cup water, bottled   **juice of ½ lemon**
1 avocado   **pinch of vegetable salt**

Cut pineapple in small cubes. Add water, avocado, honey, lemon and salt. Blend in blender until smooth and serve at once. (Use for dessert or breakfast.) Serves 4 or 6.

AVOCADO DRESSING

1 avocado   **juice of ½ lemon**
1 papaya   **1 teaspoon natural mineral salt**
juice of 2 oranges

Blend all ingredients in a blender. Use with fruit salad. Serves 6.

PINEAPPLE DRESSING

6 ounces apricot-kernel oil
5 ounces honey
1 pineapple cut in small cubes

12 ounces carrot juice
1 avocado
½ teaspoon Spike

Blend all ingredients. Serves 6.

LEMON-HONEY DRESSING

Stir together ¼ cup lemon juice, 2 tablespoons honey, 2 table-spoons apricot-kernel oil, ½ teaspoon celery seed and ½ teaspoon Spike. Serves 4 to 6.

SALAD DRESSING

2 teaspoons guava concentrate
2 teaspoons Poco-V
1 tablespoon saltmarsh vinegar
1 teaspoon B amino
1 teaspoon B minerals
2 tablespoons M.P. oil

2 tablespoons lemon juice
several sprinkles yerba santa
several sprinkles oregano
several sprinkles elderblossom
   (with fruit salad)
several sprinkles tru organic seasoning

You may add one or more of the following: Egg, tomato paste, grated cheese, vege-nut soup, fresh chopped garlic, fresh ground pepper, vege-sea salt.

᭥§ SUGGESTIONS FOR BLENDER ৪ঌ

PARSLEY DRESSING

6 ounces sunflower oil
20 ounces water (bottled)
5 ounces honey
3½ ounces lemon juice

1 cup parsley, pressed down
2 teaspoons sweet basil
mineral seasoning salt to taste
1 cup avocado

Blend well. Serves 6.

TOMATO DRESSING

6 ounces olive oil
1½ ounces lemon juice
5 ounces honey
4 cups tomatoes

mineral seasoning salt to taste
1 teaspoon sweet basil
¼ teaspoon oregano
2 tablespoons tahini (optional)

Blend well. Serves 6.

GREEN BELL PEPPER DRESSING

6 ounces apricot-kernel oil
2 cups fresh pineapple, cut up
2 cups water
2 cups green pepper, chopped
1 cup avocado

5 ounces honey
1½ teaspoons mineral salt
1 teaspoon sweet basil
1½ teaspoons vanilla

Blend well. Serves 6.

GREEN PEPPER RELISH

1 cup finely chopped celery
1½ cups chopped green pepper

½ cup scallions
1 cup diced tomatoes

Mix all together in a wooden bowl and serve with following dressing: blend in a blender, ½ cup oil, 2 teaspoons honey, juice of 1 lemon, 2 teaspoons mineral salt and 1 avocado. Serves 3.

TOMATO-OKRA SOUP

4 cups tomatoes
1 tablespoon okra
1 scant cup raisins
2 tablespoons apricot-kernel oil
1 tablespoon horseradish, grated fresh

1 teaspoon sweet basil
¾ cup celery leaves and stalks
natural mineral salt to taste
    and a dash of Spike

Add water to cover all. Blend well; eat raw. Makes 4 cups.

ASPARAGUS SOUP

1 pound fresh asparagus
1 celery stalk
a sprig parsley
dash of oregano, dash thyme

2 tablespoons apricot-kernel oil
1 tablespoon almond meal
  or ground nuts
1 teaspoon of Spike

Blend two to three minutes. Makes 4-5 cups.

MUSTARD GREEN AND CELERY SOUP

Into a 48-ounce blender, place the following in order given: 2 cups fresh corn, fill to the 28-ounce level with chopped, shredded mustard greens. Add chopped celery leaves and stalks to fill to the 48-ounce level, 2 tablespoons apricot-kernel oil, or any other vegetable oil, natural mineral salt to taste, 1 teaspoon honey. Blend ten to fifteen minutes. A nice peppery taste resembling the nippiness of watercress. Makes 4-6 cups.

WALNUT CORN SOUP

Put into a blender the following: ¾ cup hot water; ¼ cup broken walnut meats; 2 cups fresh corn; 1 teaspoon honey; 1 cup chopped celery; 2 green pepper rings, cut up; ¼ teaspoon mineral salt; 1 teaspoon apricot-kernel oil, small pinch of capsicum. Blend and heat to serving temperature. Makes 2 cups.

GRAPE SLAW WITH BANANA DRESSING

¼ cup mayonnaise
2 teaspoons prepared yellow mustard
2 tablespoons lemon juice
2 medium ripe bananas

4 cups finely shredded green cabbage
  (packed down)
2 teaspoons natural mineral salt
2 cups seedless grapes, halved

In a large mixing bowl, stir together mayonnaise, mustard and lemon juice. Slice in bananas; mash fine with dressing. Add cabbage and sprinkle with salt; mix well. Fold in grapes. Salad may be served right away or may be chilled for several hours. Serves 6.

PEAR GRENADINE SALAD

1½ tablespoons unflavored gelatin
¼ cup cold water
1 cup grenadine
½ cup pineapple juice

¼ cup lemon juice
¼ cup orange juice
4 pears halved and slightly precooked

Soften gelatin in cold water for five minutes. Bring grenadine, pineapple, lemon and orange juices to boiling point. Dissolve gelatin in hot liquid. Pour into 6-cup mold over the pears. Refrigerate until set. Unmold onto salad greens. Set upright around mold. Decorate molded salad with cream cheese softened slightly with cream. Serves 8.

FRUIT BOWL

4 fresh pears
2 medium oranges
16 prunes (soaked)

1 banana
shredded lettuce
1 pint cottage cheese

Halve and core pears. Pare and slice oranges, pit prunes. Peel and quarter banana lengthwise. Fill bottom of shallow wooden bowl with shredded lettuce. Arrange cottage cheese in center with fruit around it. Serve with dressing. Serves 4.

FRUITED COLE SLAW

1 cup sliced fresh apricots
⅔ cup grapefruit sections
2 cups shredded cabbage
¼ cup thick sour cream

1 tablespoon vinegar
¼ teaspoon mineral salt
2 tablespoons honey

Dice apricots and prepare grapefruit. Combine with cabbage. Blend together remaining ingredients and pour over mixture. Toss lightly until well mixed. Serves 4.

MINT CHUTNEY

Mint, green grapes, salt, pomegranate seeds and vinegar. First chop mint very fine, then grind the rest of the ingredients, adding vinegar to taste.

HUNZA GRAPE VINEGAR

Wash grapes well and place in a wooden bowl for seven days. Then mash grapes with hands, strain through a cheese cloth. Place the juice in a glass bottle and seal well, letting it stand for forty days.

HUNZA GRAPE WINE

Same as above, but let stand for about ninety days.

THE MONO DIET

The Mono diet means consuming only one particular food during the whole day. Usually it is done with fruits or vegetables. However, it is advisable to go on a Mono diet when fruits are in season, and one can secure them freshly picked from the garden. The average amount of fruits consumed during such periods varies from two to four pounds per day. It can be done with solid fruit or juices, in case of juices three to six pints per day, freshly squeezed at home.

As a rule three meals are taken, and some water can be consumed in between meals—preferably bottled spring water! There is no rule for how long one can stay on a Mono diet. However, three to four days are perfectly safe. It can be done once a week for instance. These suggestions are from Dr. Maxwell O. Garten's book, *The Dynamics of Vibrant Health.*

A sample menu for a Mono diet routine: *First Day:* 1 to 2 quarts of freshly prepared apple juice, or 2 pounds of raw apples. Apples are to be washed thoroughly and chewed.

Second Day: 1 to 2 quarts of freshly squeezed orange juice, or three pounds of oranges. Oranges are to be eaten without seeds or skins.

Third Day: ½ to 1½ quarts of freshly-made celery juice or its equivalent of fresh celery stalks.

This can be done with all kinds of fruits or vegetables.

The Hunza generally eat a Mono diet menu. Their foods don't vary too much.

WHOLE KERNEL GRAINS

Wheat, barley, oats, rye, brown rice and millet can all be considered as coming from the same family. If grown on a well-nourished soil with nothing taken out in milling, all these foods are rich in valuable nutrients and should be added to your daily diet.

The grain should be soaked overnight and next day brought just below the boiling point. Then continue to cook in a double boiler. It makes an excellent cereal for breakfast.

LENTILS

These are a good source of iron and other minerals. Vitamins A and E are generously supplied.

GARBANZOS (also called CHICK PEAS)

They are said to be rich in vitamins and minerals. Garbanzos require a long cooking process. They can be sprouted and eaten raw.

SOY BEANS

Soy beans are very high in nutritional value. The soy bean serves in many capacities such as providing protein for the making of cheese, milk, bakery goods, etc.

CAROB POWDER

This is an excellent natural food resembling chocolate in flavor and appearance. It can be used in cold milk, or various desserts can be made from it—any recipe that calls for chocolate can be substituted by carob powder. Among the early Christians it was known as St. John's bread. An excellent food for children instead of candies or sugars. Cora-coa is a ready-made carob drink.

SUNFLOWER SEEDS

There are many reasons why sunflower seeds should be eaten. Nature protects these seeds with a shell and the seed itself loses very little of its food value after it has been taken off stem.

It is eaten raw. We need more raw foods in our daily diet. These seeds are said to be rich in protein, oil and especially in Vitamin B. Many experiments are being conducted with sunflower seeds and new discoveries as to their nutrient composition are being made all the time.

A handful of seeds a few times a day whenever you feel hungry might help you keep your weight down. They should be well chewed.

OILS

All vegetable oils contain the unsaturated fatty acids—especially linoleic acid, which is important for good health. At least 2 to 3 tablespoons should be added to your diet daily, either mixed in your salad or taken as is. I take it with my milk using the following proportions: 1 tablespoonful of multipurpose oil (more or less), a combination of various oils, with 5 tablespoons of whole milk. Mix it well and drink it either before going to bed or three hours after your last meal, or an hour before your breakfast.

The combination of these various oils provide a better balance of ingredients for body fat. People who use such a balance of oils, notice that digestion and bowel action may improve. Your doctor will advise you as to the total calorie intake you should have daily. The Hunza people eat a great deal of their apricot-kernel oil (see the discussion in Chapter Nine) and they are all slim. In addition, they have fine skin, beautiful hair and lovely complexions.

Quoting from an article Changing Aspects of Nutrition, from *Modern Nutrition* by J. D. Walters, M.D., who says: "During the past two decades, considerable attention has been focused on nutrition, especially the phases concerned with vitamins, amino acids, and minerals. More recently evidence has been presented that definite relationships exist between these, as well as between endocrines and minerals and amino acids and unsaturated fatty acids."

I am fond of apricot-kernel oil, but there are many others: safflower, poppyseed, sunflower, soybean, corn, wheat germ, cottonseed, sesame, avocado, peanut, flaxseed and olive. But no matter which oil you use, make sure it is not rancid, and protect it from light and air. A walnut oil is also produced now.

POWDERED SKIM MILK

Powdered skim milk is a nourishing beverage and added to your regular skim milk greatly increases its food value. It can be made in the following manner: mix ½ cup of powdered skim milk into a quart of whole or skimmed fluid milk. Whole milk is for those who aren't worried about additional calories. Powdered skim milk, rich in proteins, increases the intake of your proteins daily, and is practically free from fat, but rich in calcium and other vitamins. Another advantage is that since it comes in a dry powder form, it can be stored easily. Remember to keep it away from light and air, just as any other food, to preserve the nutrient contents.

This powdered milk can be added to many of your meals by using it in custards, soups and sauces as well as in baking of breads, muffins, etc., without changing the original recipe.

SPROUTING

The Hunza people sprout the following seeds which convert starches into proteins: soybeans, alfalfa seeds, lentils, green peas, lima beans, whole-wheat kernels and barley.

The preparation of sprouting is simple. You need a mason or a glass baking dish. Put into it a handful of desired seeds and soak them overnight in lukewarm water. Cover it tightly with a kitchen towel. The best thing is to cover it with a dish exactly the same size. Next morning place a strainer over the open end and pour off the water. Repeat this procedure twice a day for at least two or three days. Make sure that the seeds are kept from packing as they begin to swell. The seeds will burst open and little sprouts will appear. Then the dish can be placed on the window, where the sunlight can get to them. The little sprouts that emerge from the seeds will then have a healthy green color, and sunlight gives the seeds a special pleasant flavor.

At this stage they are ready to be eaten. Pluck the sprouts and use them with your salads or sprinkle with lemon juice and some of your favorite vegetable oil. They are delicious and quite nourishing.

If you consider sprouting a complicated job, then pick up a prepared package at your health-food store. Sunflower and sesame seeds can also be sprouted.

HUNZA YOGURT

Yogurt in Hunza is made by a very simple method. The people of Hunza pour milk into a pot, cover it with a heavy lid and leave it overnight in a warm place. The following day the creamy top from the milk is removed and then beaten into butter. The remaining thickened milk is served as a drink.

The Hunzas use yogurt frequently, serving it with their meals as a beverage and cooking it with their various foods.

YOGURT AT ANY TIME

1 cup yogurt   1 teaspoon of Brewer's yeast
1 teaspoon of wheat germ

Mix all ingredients well. Top with sunflower seeds or sunflower seeds meal and berries or any other fruit.

HUNZA COTTAGE CHEESE

Goat's milk or cow's milk is soured overnight by leaving it in a warm place, covered with a lid. The following day it is heated over a low fire. When the milk curdles it is removed from the stove and poured into a muslin bag. After it is drained the curdles form the cottage cheese. The drained juice is served with meals.

HERB TEAS

The Hunzakuts drink various herb teas instead of coffee or regular teas. They grow a variety of herbs in their gardens and dry them for the winter season. We also have a variety of herb teas in our country, and some of them are delicious. The most popular are peppermint, alfalfa, papaya, oats and many others. Served cold or hot with lemon juice and honey, they make a very refreshing drink.

FRUIT JUICES

My daily diet includes at least one glass of both—fruit and vegetable juice. The greatest benefit of these juices is derived when they are fresh.

The juice can be extracted from almost every vegetable including their green tops. Popular vegetables are carrots, celery, beets and cucumbers, but there are many others which are also very nutritious. For instance, potato and cabbage juices are also excellent.

Fruit juices, such as apple, apricot, pineapple, pear, coconut, papaya, etc., are a delightful treat between meals, and will help control your appetite.

An excellent pep drink can be prepared from any of these juices, enriched with a teaspoonful of plain gelatin. Wheat germ, Brewer's yeast and, if you prefer it sweet, some honey or molasses can also be added. Mix well in your blender.

✺§ DRINKS MADE IN A BLENDER ℘

CAROB MILK DRINK

2 tablespoons dry skim-milk powder
1 pint of fluid skim milk

1 tablespoon of carob extract
few drops of vanilla (optional)

Mix well. For best results mix in blender. This is an excellent between-meal drink.

MOLASSES DRINK

1 pint fluid skim milk
2 tablespoons dry skim milk powder

2 teaspoons unsulphured molasses

Mix well in blender.

PINEAPPLE DRINK

2 cups cubed fresh pineapple
1 tablespoon wheat germ

1 tablespoon powdered skim milk
1 teaspoon honey

To enrich it add one tablespoon of a commercial protein powder. Blend all together. If it doesn't blend too well add some pineapple juice or bottled water.

STRAWBERRY DRINK

1 glass of skim milk
1 tablespoon dry skim-milk powder
1 tablespoon wheat germ

1 tablespoon Brewer's yeast
1 teaspoon honey

Mix thoroughly in blender and add 1 cup of sliced strawberries. You may prefer to chill this drink and then top it with almond or nut meal.

◆§ NATURAL BALANCED DRINK MADE IN A BLENDER ð◆

2 teaspoons guava concentrate
1 tablespoon PAP fruit concentrate
   (peach, apple, plum)
1 tablespoon ampro (organs)
2 teaspoons wheat germ oil (virgin)
1 tablespoon M.P. oil
2 teaspoons Tastee dessert
1 tablespoon orange and yeast

2 teaspoons malted almonds—vary
   with malted coconut or malted
   almonds and cashews
2 teaspoons whole date and pit
1 tablespoon baby veal liver
2 teaspoons enzyme calcium
1 or 2 raw fertile eggs
1 or 2 glasses raw certified whole milk

add any other fruit in season

Blend thoroughly and serve. It is almost a complete meal. Refrigerate the balance for use as a raw pudding. Herb aroma tea, or garden treet tea may be used instead of milk.

(This is the famous recipe of the Sunshine Valley. You can find the necessary ingredients in your diet store.)

MORNING PEP COCKTAIL

1 or 2 egg yolks   1 glass of fresh orange juice

Blend well. The same drink can be enriched with 1 teaspoon of Brewer's yeast and 1 tablespoon of wheat germ.

PAPAYA JUICE

If papaya is in concentrated form, dilute according to instructions on can, add 1 teaspoon of gelatin (natural) and stir well. It is a good source of protein. Drink in the morning before breakfast or between meals.

PROTEIN DRINK

2 tablespoons protein powder
1 glass of liquid (choose your favorite fruit juice)

Mix the liquid with the protein. Skim milk can be used instead of the juice. Blend until smooth. Add yogurt and honey to taste. Any of the commercial proteins can be used. For richer flavor top it with fresh fruit in season.

Imagination and experiments will lead you to the proper combinations. All you need do is to supply your kitchen with the necessary gadgets, such as:

A *liquidizer blender*, which includes many wonders in one machine: it chops, whips and grinds all in one.

A *modern juicer*, which doesn't need to be too large for a small family. It is easy to keep clean at all times.

Good *cooking utensils*, which will preserve the value of your food.

Another gadget which I consider a "must" in every kitchen is a *stainless-steel vegetable and fruit shredder*. You simply cannot enjoy a salad without having your carrots, beets or celery shredded properly. Besides, shredding makes vegetables look much more appetizing. It has another good point—your salad is prepared quickly, which preserves all the nutrients.

No doubt there are many more useful utensils to simplify the preparation of meals, so when you shop next time in your natural-diet food shop, make a point to ask for them.

*   *   *

For any additional information drop me a note and I will be happy to be of service and share with you my favorites. Write to Renée Taylor, P.O. Box 995, Beverly Hills, California.

A HUNZA PICTURE ALBUM

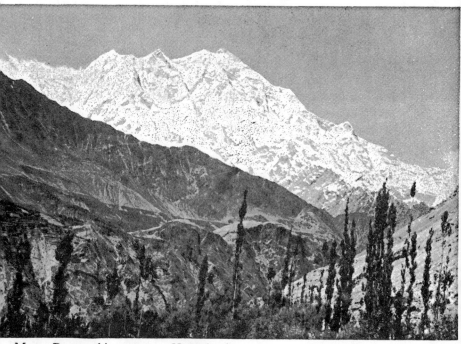

Mount Rapaposhi towers over Hunzaland —
25,560 feet high — and is covered with snow
the year round.

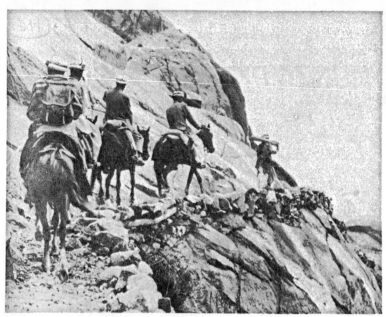

A typical mountain trail into Hunzaland,
barely wide enough for two horses to pass
one another.

Volley ball Hunza style.
Participants are over seventy years old.

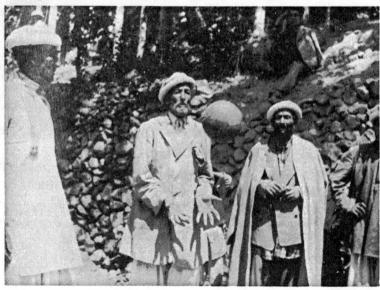

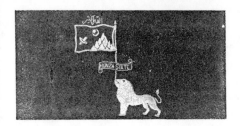

The Hunza flag with insignia.

The Mir, wearing his ceremonial robes,
presides at the daily court session
on the roof of the old fort.

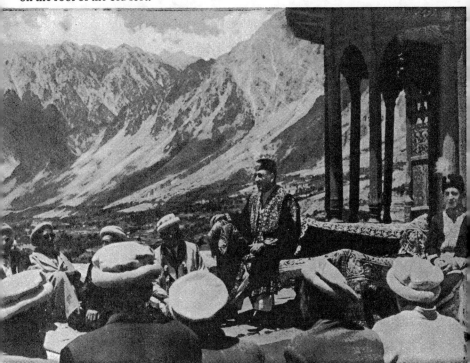

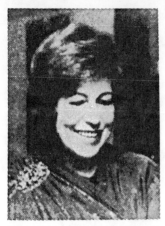

The author, Renée Taylor, who has made many
trips to Hunzaland.

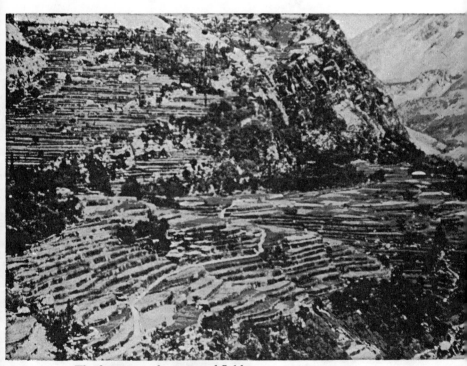

The famous garden terraced fields.
Since every speck of land must be utilized,
fields stretch high up into the mountains.

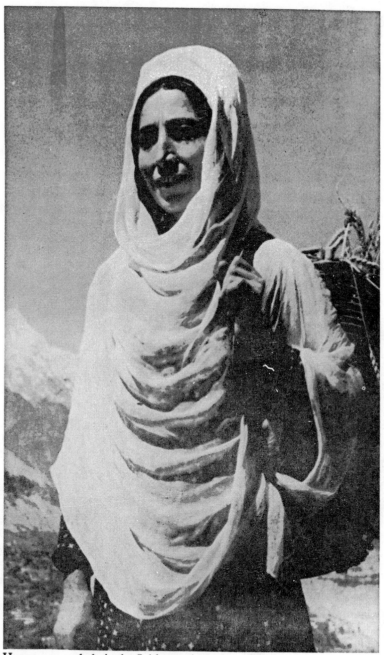

Hunza women help in the fields wearing
protective scarves — but the real heavy work
is reserved for the men.

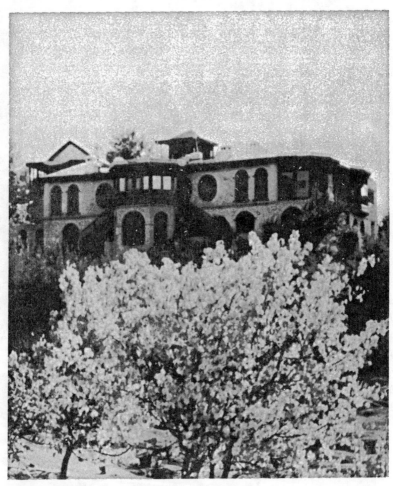

The new palace of the Mir, or ruling head of the
Hunzakuts, has almost every modern convenience.

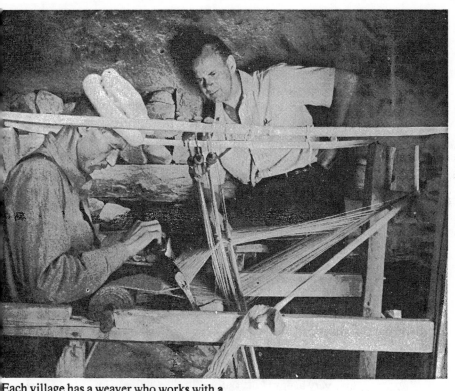

Each village has a weaver who works with a
handmade loom to provide his community with the
fabric from which clothes are made. M.J. Nobbs,
sponsor of the author's first Hunza expedition,
is the interested watcher.

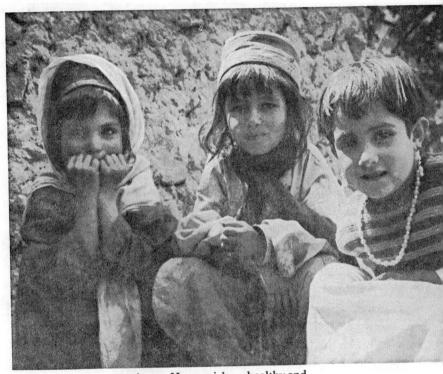

Three very happy Hunza girls — healthy and
"very obedient" (according to the author).

II.

Minerals, Enzymes and Food for Thought

Hunza food is superior in nourishment because its essential values are not lost between the soil and the table.

On the other hand, we know what happens to our own foods through storage of foods in the warehouse, through transport to the market in freezers, through taking the fruits off the trees before they have a chance to ripen, through peeling the skin off our vegetables and fruits (because of the chemical sprays) and finally through prolonged cooking.

It may come as a surprise to the average housewife to know how much of the food so beautifully displayed in a supermarket is grown in poor soil and sprayed with poisonous chemicals. By no means can such food be considered as nourishing as food growing in soil similar to the Hunza valley. Thus our bodies slowly fall behind par, and strength and energy begin to fail us. When we do not get the right amount of protein, carbohydrates, fat, vitamins and minerals, the cellular structure of the body breaks down.

For instance, spinach has in addition to protein, fat, carbohydrates and vitamins, the minerals calcium, phosphates, magnesium and iron. The Hunzakuts eat large quantities of spinach. It is practically served with every meal. But spinach grown in mineral-poor soil is virtually worthless.

Many of us fail to understand the importance of a balanced mineral supply in the building and maintaining of robust health. The average person knows more about vitamins than about minerals. Balanced nutrition demands that an adequate supply of all the essential minerals be present in the body, as these minerals work as a team with vitamins in rebuilding the body cells. Vitamins and minerals are dependent on one another. Lack of one or more of either minerals or vitamins may cause the loss of many valuable nutrients in the body.

The body is composed of sixteen or seventeen known minerals, all of which are found in the soil.

Calcium Essential for good bone structure and strong teeth. It is also important for calm nerves and for maintaining good muscle tone. Although four grams of calcium should be consumed daily, sometimes less than one gram is taken into the body with the usual diet. The best natural sources of calcium are fresh fruits and vegetables (particularly the green leafy vegetables); whole grains; dairy products, including milk in all forms and cheeses; nuts; dark or blackstrap molasses; soybeans and soybean flour, and bone meal. In order for calcium to be properly absorbed into the system, hydrochloric acid must be present in the stomach to hold the mineral in solution for absorption in the small intestines. Sodium is also valuable to aid in the assimilation of calcium.

Calcium may be taken between meals to supplement the diet. It is available in capsule, tablet or powdered form, but is best assimilated when adequate Vitamin C, Vitamin D and phosphorus are present. Vitamin F will help to increase the calcium ions in the blood and the calcium in soft tissue. Eating raw celery will supply sufficient sodium in the system when calcium is taken in large quantities.

Phosphorus Equally essential for good tooth and bone structure as well as for healthy brain tissue and nervous system. Phosphorus is found in the structure of each cell nucleus. Phosphorus also assists in the maintenance of the acid-alkaline balance in the system. Calcium is necessary for the proper assimilation of phosphorus. Both should be present simultaneously in the diet. When there is not enough calcium present to combine with phosphorus, it is lost through the kidneys. Fortunately, most of our foods contain phosphorus in large quantities: such as whole grains, dairy products, eggs, meats, legumes and nuts. And nearly all fruits and vegetables contain some phosphorus. There is seldom a deficiency of this mineral in a good normal diet.

Iron Essential for building red blood cells, which bring oxygen to the cells and take away carbon dioxide. A deficiency of iron, and consequently a deficiency of red blood cells, causes anemia in varying degrees. There is a surprisingly high number of women in the United States who have been found to be anemic or bordering on anemia.

Iron is best assimilated into the system in a natural organic form. However, assimilation of iron and other minerals depends on a sufficient amount of acid in the stomach. Including the intake of vinegar with your meals (good vinegar, aged one or more years) will increase the acidity in your stomach for better mineral utilization.

Iodine Such a tiny amount of this mineral is needed in the body that there is no excuse for anyone to be deficient in iodine. But that tiny amount is so important it is better to include an ample supply in the daily diet than to take a chance of being undersupplied. Lack of iodine causes many deficiency symptoms, such as goiter, unbalanced fat deposits and even the appearance of stupidity. It has been said that a tiny amount of this mineral can make the difference between a genius and an imbecile. The thyroid gland, located at the base of the throat, regulates the body metabolism and requires small amounts of iodine daily to function properly. Iodine is not toxic in food form, and any iodine not used will be discarded. All sea foods, both animal and vegetable, are rich in iodine. Cod-liver oil is an excellent source, and dehydrated sea kelp and dulce offers a wonderful source in concentrated form. Table salt, if used, should always be the raw sea salt. Plants grown in soils rich in iodine are also a good source.

Copper Necessary for the proper utilization of iron in the body and the prevention of anemia. The best sources are sea foods, liver, molasses, green leafy vegetables, soy products, egg yolk, whole grains and fruits, particularly dried fruits. Apricots are especially rich in copper and iron. The Hunzakuts are blessed with a rich intake of copper from apricots.

Sodium Keeps the body in acid-alkaline balance and is neces sary to keep calcium in solution. Salt (sodium chloride) is the principal source of sodium, although this mineral is found in vegetables and muscle meats. Celery is particularly rich in sodium. Heat stroke and muscle cramps may result from a deficiency of sodium. Salt tablets are taken during hot weather by those engaged in hard physical labor or sports to prevent a deficiency because of loss through perspiration.

Potassium   Important for body growth and, like sodium, it functions as a balancer. Sodium and potassium in combination help the body cells absorb nourishment from the bloodstream. Potassium also assists in ridding the cells of waste matter. Dark or blackstrap molasses, dulce, kelp, leafy green vegetables, whole grains, fruits and almonds are excellent sources of potassium. However, it is largely lost when foods are refined or when vegetable-cooking water is discarded. Poor soil in which the plant grows could easily create a deficiency of this important mineral.

Magnesium   Necessary to maintain mineral balance in the body and the elasticity of the muscles. It is an aid in the digestion and elimination of foods. The best source is green leafy vegetables. Chlorophyll, which gives the green coloring to plants, is rich in magnesium. Like potassium, the water in which vegetables are cooked should be used in some manner, otherwise the mineral will be lost. Whole-grain breads and cereals contain magnesium, but it is not found in the refined products.

Manganese   This mineral gives strength to the tissues and bones and protects the inner lining of the heart and blood vessels. Although its exact action in the body is little understood, manganese is necessary to human growth and health. It is related to the use of calcium and phosphorus and is found in the bones. Green leaves and whole grains contain a generous supply of manganese when they are grown on good soil. Manganese is a great activator of the enzymes in our system and nothing happens in the body without an enzyme being involved. Enzymes run our system.

Chlorine   A constituent of the acid in the gastric juice in the stomach. It also aids in the purification and cleansing of the system.

Fluorine   Helps build strong bones and tooth enamel and also builds up the resistance of the body.

Carbon, Hydrogen, Oxygen, Nitrogen   Of all the elements that go to make up the cells of the human body, carbon, hydrogen, oxygen and nitrogen are by far the most abundant, as they are the essential elements of the organic foodstuffs.

Few of us realize the importance of these minerals. For example, if your body lacked iodine for any appreciable time, you would be likely to suffer from goiter. If it lacked iron, you would probably develop anemia or liver trouble, your skin and hair would pale and become harsh and your body would show signs of emaciation. If your body contained no cobalt, the number of red corpuscles in your body would be reduced, glandular activity would be lessened and you would become listless and lethargic.

Many doctors and nutrition specialists believe that a deficiency of silver will cause diseased tonsils; that a deficiency of magnesium will cause nervous disorders; a deficiency of zinc will cause thyroid troubles, and so on.

Despite the knowledge of the injurious effects which deficiencies in these minerals can cause, the average person seldom gives a thought to his body's requirements. Not until he becomes sick or indisposed does he start purchasing vitamins and minerals, either as a result of reading advertisements or on a doctor's prescription.

Preferably, minerals and vitamins should be obtained from our foods. However, since foods are often deficient in essential minerals and vitamins due to poor soil and unfavorable marketing conditions, it is almost a necessity to supplement our diets with bottled natural minerals and vitamins to avoid the hazards of an under-supply. There are many good brands of natural minerals and vitamins on the market.

ENZYMES

Enzymes are delicate lifelike substances found in all living cells, whether vegetable or animal. Their presence and strength can be determined only by means of refined tests. Enzymes break up into small molecules: proteins, fats, starches, maltose, sucrose, lactose and cellulose.

Life could not exist without enzymes. They digest all food and make it small enough to pass through the minute pores of the intestine into the blood. They are thought to rebuild the prepared food into muscle, nerve, bone or gland. Enzymes assist in storing excess food in the liver or muscles for future use.

Nature puts enzymes into all food together with vitamins, minerals, fats, proteins, carbohydrates and water. However, all of this food is completely indigestible until enzymes work on it and break down complex foods into simpler substances, which the blood-stream can then absorb.

There is an enzyme to help build phosphorus into bone and nerve. Another enzyme helps fix iron in the red blood cells. Enzymes can change protein into fat or sugar. Enzymes change carbohydrates into fat and enzymes change fats into carbohydrates.

Enzymes perform in a few minutes chemical transformations that are impossible to perform in laboratories. Without the help of enzymes we could stuff ourselves with food and still literally starve. Although enzymes are just as important to good nutrition as vitamins and minerals, they are not nearly as delicate. The length of life of an enzyme depends on temperature. When enzymes are subjected to boiling temperature for even a few minutes, they are completely destroyed. Boiling potatoes, meat or leafy vegetables in water causes a destruction of enzymes.

Enzymes in the dormant state, as found in dry seeds, retain their activity for hundreds of years. They have been found in rice stored for one hundred years. Several investigators have found enzymes in Egyptian mummies three thousand years old. One scientist found them in the flesh of ancient mammoths about fifty thousand years old. Carcasses of these prehistoric elephants are found occasionally in Siberia, buried in graves of ice and snow, the perpetual cold having maintained them in a well-preserved condition. Enzymes are preserved indefinitely when dried to a powder at blood heat, also by extreme cold.

Raw liver is a good source of certain enzymes before they are lost in the frying pan. Sun-ripened fruits and vegetables are rich in enzymes. The sun causes the enzymes to function, as they need warmth and moisture. But there is a basic difference between the warmth of the sun (natural warmth) and the boiling process over a fire during prolonged cooking. Therefore it is absolutely essential to cook with utensils that require no water, just the natural moisture of the food and the least amount of heat.

In the manufacturing and cooking of food, certain substances are killed because of extensive heat. And since enzymes are found in the glands, organs, muscles and fluids of the body, they are necessary to carry on normal functioning. Without them we would die instantly.

To go even further, without the enzymes, seeds could not grow, leaves could not change their colors, nothing could exist, as enzymes must be present to make things grow and live. Every time we take a breath, we draw energy from these storage batteries which nature provided for our activity.

The digestive juices which are secreted in the mouth, stomach and small intestine change food into products that can be used to meet the demands of the body. Each of these digestive secretions has enzymes in it, and it is the enzymes that change the food from one form to another. If you chew a piece of bread for a minute, you will note that it gradually becomes sweet. The body cannot utilize the starch which is in the bread, but it can absorb some of the sugar. Therefore the enzyme action in the saliva immediately begins to transform the starch into a product which can be utilized and stored in the body.

As we grow older the quota of enzymes in our body diminishes and eventually we die. In other words, we are as old as our enzymes. As long as we have sufficient enzymes in our stomach to digest the food we eat, we keep the body functioning normally.

Scientific tests in older people have shown that the body may tire of producing its own enzymes year after year, especially if a constant overdraw is experienced. Body enzymes in living things grow weaker and weaker as time goes on. And aging causes the skin to wrinkle and shrivel, hair to thin, muscles to sag and eyes to lose their sparkle.

Uncooked, unprocessed food can give you exogenous enzymes. Endogenous enzymes are those produced by the body. If more exogenous enzymes—derived from raw foods—are consumed, fewer endogenous enzymes will be needed. That means less wear and tear on your tissues.

The story of the enzymes once again proves the relationship between the good health and long life of the Hunza people and their diet—which consists largely of natural uncooked foods, including fruits and vegetables in an unaltered state from soil to table.

Here are a few foods which could very well be added daily to our regular diet to enrich the intake of minerals, vitamins, proteins, enzymes and other ingredients so essential to our good health.

NUTS

Nuts—almonds, coconuts, pecans, walnuts, beechnuts, hazelnuts, etc.—are an excellent source of protein and fat. They are the fruits of trees, bushes and plants. They are loaded with phosphoric acid, potash and magnesia, while lacking sodium, lime and chlorine. Thus nuts should be balanced with fruits and vegetables rich in sodium—such as green leafy vegetables. In combination with salads made with raw fruits and vegetables, nuts help make a complete meal.

Almonds have been rated much higher in Vitamins E and F, as well as A, B, C, D and G, than have other nuts. They are also high in protein and free from purines and other toxic agents. Eating almonds daily would enrich your diet with additional nutrients. Nut butters are being manufactured more and more and are a good source of fat and oil, especially for growing children. But be sure of the quality—most of the commercial nut butters are made from overroasted and sometimes heavily salted nuts, which destroys some of its valuable properties. Most *peanut* butters are mixed with hydrogenated oils to prevent the oil from separating. Hydrogenation destroys the food value of the oil.

Coconut is another source of essential life elements. It is low in protein but high in fat. The water of the coconut is very healthful but too rich in calories for most of us, so be careful not to drink too much. The meat of the nut can be grated and mixed with various foods. It can also be made into coconut milk or juice. Both are delicious. To make milk, grate fresh coconut with a plastic grater and squeeze through a cloth, then add coconut water drained from the fruit or add fresh bottled water.

Papaya

Papaya is a tasty fruit especially rich in enzymes which, as we know, greatly aid digestion. It is also rich in Vitamins A and C. The Spaniards were the first to learn the value of this fruit, then Professor R. H. Chittenden of Yale University confirmed the nutritional value of papaya.

The essential characteristic of papaya is its digestive ferment known as *papain*, extracted from both the juice and the latex which flow from incisions made in the skin while the fruit is still green. This is made into a commercial papain. The digestive property of papain works in acid, alkaline or neutral solutions. It helps to break down proteins, starches and fat, and aids in their digestion.

Papaya should be eaten with every meal if possible. In the tropical countries, where papaya grows in abundance, the natives indulge in this fruit in large quantities. When I visited Mexico, papaya was served with every meal. Also in Honolulu, where I was spending my Christmas holidays, I devoured large quantities of golden, ripe papaya, abstaining from other foods. I never felt better.

Papaya is being used in the manufacture of new, natural cosmetics to aid in activating the properties of skin nourishment. Some tooth powders also contain papain for digesting food particles. Eating part of the papaya seeds is recommended, too, and after you become accustomed to their flavor they are quite palatable.

If fresh papaya is not available, you will always find frozen papaya from Hawaii or fresh pulp in containers. These are good substitutes for the fresh fruit.

My own diet includes a fresh papaya daily. Living in California I am able to buy them in large quantities.

LECITHIN

Lecithin is found in many oils and foods; however, the concentrated sources which you buy in a jar are extracted from soybean oil. It is said to enhance fat metabolism and lipide transport, acting as a dissolving agent with powers to break fat and cholesterol into small particles which are then able to pass into the tissues. Lecithin should be included with each meal. The dry, or granular, form may be taken in fruit or vegetable juices or sprinkled on salads. It also comes in liquid form or in capsules.

HONEY

Honey has a high sugar content—dextrose, sucrose, glucose and levulose. Dextrose is quickly absorbed into the bloodstream and is a quick source of energy. Sucrose is the form of sugar found in sugarcane. Levulose, the queen of all sugars, digests slowly and thus gives us energy lasting for several hours, and does not overload the pancreas by dumping too much sugar into the bloodstream at one time.

Honey contains an abundant supply of minerals and trace elements, without which tissue regeneration cannot take place. It also contains vitamins and enzymes, ascorbic acid (Vitamin C), thiamin, riboflavin and other members of the Vitamin B-Complex group.

The Ancient Greeks provided for meager days by storing honey. Hippocrates included honey in his diet every day throughout his life and gave it to his patients for better health. Although honey is one of the oldest foods in existence, we are learning more about its health-giving qualities as time goes on. For instance, athletes will resort to honey during the period of training.

Honey may help to produce sleep if taken before going to bed. In choosing your favorite flavors, look for a dark color and a natural unstrained honey. The darker the color the greater the amount of mineral elements, vitamins and enzymes. Include honey in your diet daily and try to substitute it for sugar as much as possible.

Occasionally during my fasts—at least once a year—I would take a spoonful of honey when I felt tired. It was amazing how quickly my energy returned. It is a good food for busy Americans.

WHEAT GERM AND WHEAT-GERM OIL

The inner part of the wheat kernel—called the *endosperm*—consists mostly of starch and small amounts of protein. It contains almost no vitamins or minerals. White flour is made from this part of the kernel and then enriched with vitamins, minerals and proteins.

The *embryo*, or wheat germ, is the life-giving part from which the wheat plant sprouts and is one of the richest known sources of the B and E vitamins. It also contains valuable proteins and fats. During the production of large quantities of flour, the germ has to be removed to prevent it from becoming rancid. Thus we are given the legacy in the form of wheat germ and wheat-germ oil.

Scientists consider wheat germ and wheat-germ oil a wonderful addition to the daily diet, providing man with a food element which gives added endurance under physical stress. Experiments with athletes at the Physical Fitness Laboratory of the University of Illinois showed fitness scores were higher with wheat germ or wheat-germ oil added to the diet than with exercise alone.

The Hunzakuts eat the whole grain with every meal and, as we know, they don't remove anything from it. In this way they get the full benefit from eating their homemade bread and cereals.

Wheat-germ oil may be added to your salad dressing and the wheat-germ kernels may be sprinkled over salads, cereals or soup. You can eat it with cottage cheese, with yogurt and with fresh-fruit salad. There are many ways of using wheat germ in your cooking: in breads, muffins, hotcakes and waffles, and in hamburger patties and meat loaf. All oils are perishable; wheat-germ oil is no exception. Vacuum-packing of wheat germ in can or jar prevents oxygenation or rancidity. Rancidity is detrimental to health, therefore all fats, flours and ground-up cereals should be refrigerated to retard oxygenation.

YOGURT

The great scientist Dr. Eli Metchnikoff was the first to hail the powers of yogurt. He found that the Bulgarians, great eaters of yogurt, had 1666 people over ninety years of age for each million of population, while our rate is a mere nine people over ninety per million.

Yogurt, kefir or other kinds of cultured milk supply valuable acids that greatly assist digestion and are beneficial for the friendly bacteria in the intestinal tract.

Yogurt is fermented milk that has been left standing at room temperature and allowed to sour. You can easily make it yourself. However, it needs a special yogurt culture called Bulgarious sold in health-food stores; added to the milk, it helps thicken the yogurt into a form of custard.

Yogurt is delicious, and there are many ways of eating it: as a dessert with fresh fruit, all by itself or in many recipes (see p. 100).

BREWERS' YEAST

Brewers' yeast contains almost no fat, starch or sugar and is an excellent source of protein and Vitamin B-Complex. The best way to get accustomed to the taste of yeast is to begin with one teaspoon to a large glass of fruit juice or milk and to continue to increase the amount. My favorite dish for breakfast is a generous portion of cottage cheese with powdered yeast and honey.

25 WAYS TO PROTECT YOUR HEALTH AND PROLONG YOUTHFUL VIGOR

1. Eat only if hungry, and don't confuse hunger with appetite. False appetite is a function of habit; true hunger is physiological.

2. Pass up one meal a day for a while. Americans eat too much and the average person can get along with one-half to one-third the amount of food he has been eating.

3. Chew the food thoroughly and mix it well with saliva.

4. Never eat when tired.

5. Do not take a bath immediately after eating, but before.

6. Avoid eating between meals unless you have fruit juice or fresh fruit.

7. Do not eat when you are emotionally upset.

8. Do not drink water with your food. Drink it twenty minutes before the meal or four hours after it.

9. Avoid pastries made from refined flours and hydrogenated fats.

10. Avoid soft drinks, synthetic ice creams, chocolate, etc.

11. Try to sleep at least eight hours daily. Remember, the most beneficial sleep is before midnight.

12. Sleep with your window open; shun all sleeping garments; arrange bed with head toward the north and foot end slightly raised.

13. Maintain a cheerful and positive attitude; never permit negative thoughts to linger.

14. Try to get sunshine every day on your body. (The sun is the source of all energy, and its invigorating rays will soon leave you with a renewed feeling of vitality.)

15. Breathe deeply and rhythmically; fresh air is essential to good health.

16. Walk two hours every day.

17. Always eat fresh fruits and vegetables in season, preferably raw.

18. Try the mono diet occasionally—eat only a single vegetable or fruit at a meal.

19. Use the waterless-cooking method. A set of stainless-steel waterless-cookware utensils should be used in every household. But be sure that it is a tri-ply cookware pattern, which is constructed with a heavy double-layer bottom to provide additional protection from the heat.

20. Shop regularly for vegetable oils, cider vinegar, honey, mineralized eggs, natural mineral salt and the other special ingredients suggested in the preceding recipes. They are available in your health-food store.

21. Add to your daily diet all kind of seeds—pumpkin, sesame, etc., and also almonds and other nuts.

22. Add Brewers' yeast, lecithin and wheat germ to your daily menu. (These products can be eaten with yogurt and cottage cheese, added to your salad or mixed in fruit juices.)

23. Drink milk, buttermilk, kefir or yogurt and, if it is at all possible, buy the certified kind.

24. Eat plenty of animal-organ meats, such as brain, kidney, liver, etc.

25. Every home should have a little mill and flour should be ground, as it is needed, for making bread. If this is not practical, try stone-ground flours and grains. In any case, learn to make your own bread.

26. Apricot-kernel oil is also available as a cosmetic for your skin.

12.

Fasting and Philosophy

There is a time in Hunza when there is no food to be had at any price: in the late spring before the new harvest has been gathered. Then the Hunzakuts go on an enforced fast. During this fast the digestive mechanism of the body is given a rest, the body lives on its own reserves, and old cells are eliminated. What is left constitutes the nucleus, or basis, of a new sound body.

It is true that the body requires food, but it is a false assumption when we think we receive strength only from the food we eat. The body, collectively, consists of myriads of cells, each a body in itself, complete with head and brain. This little brain of the cells is technically known as the nucleus and consists primarily of gray matter. But there is more to this dynamic little speck than that. This gray matter has the ability to store magnetic energy within itself. Thus in each and every one of our cells we can receive and store up potential cosmic energy.

If the body carries a great deal of waste material, one tires very easily and general aches and pains may be felt in any part of the body, most likely along the backbone. Along with this goes a feeling of pessimism and negativism. Our impaired and clogged body mechanism is the payment for the long years of abuse we have forced it to endure.

Many doctors support the theory of fasting. Dr. Otto Buchinger, who maintained two famous sanitoriums in Germany, is an excellent example. While still a young man he suffered not only from liver and gallbladder disorders, but also from arthritis of the knees that nearly reduced him to a cripple. A physician in the German navy, he was discharged because of his illness. Nevertheless he tried various remedies, which only offered temporary relief. One doctor suggested a water fast. Under the supervision of the doctor, he underwent a twenty-eight-day fast. The results were spectacular.

After regaining his health, Dr. Buchinger adopted the fasting routine and became a very successful physician. At seventy-eight he still felt strong and young. He said, "Through the grace of God I was permitted to see so many fine things and received such untold blessings that I owe the universe a great debt."

Fasting was practiced in northern Europe among the Druids, in America among the Indians, and throughout India, Palestine, China, Persia, Babylon, Greece and Rome. The Bible records many fasts, and advises fasters not to wear a sad countenance (Matt. 6:16) but to find pleasure in fasting and to perform one's work (Isa. 58:3).

It can be assumed that the ancients were not afraid of starving to death by missing a few meals. Among the early Christians, total fasting was practiced for one or two days each week. For two thousand years prayer and periodic fasting has been recommended by Christian dogma.

It has also been traditionally believed that fasting improves the mind and soul. Mohammed said, "Prayers lead halfway to God, fasting brings one to the doors of heaven." The famous monk and philosopher Roger Bacon (1214–1294) recommended periodic fasts. "To prevent brittleness and degeneration in old age, one should, every two or three years, submit to a rejuvenation through elimination of all used fluids by fasting and diet."

In 1724 the French physician Dr. P. Carton reported a method of the Pater Bernhard von Malra, who had astonishing success in the treatment of advanced chronic disease. Information found in Dr. Maxwell O. Garten's book, *The Dynamics of Vibrant Health*, published in 1958.

> Dr. Carton writes with enthusiasm about the periodic fast: The clinical results of fasting are noteworthy. The violence of intoxication troubles ebb off, breathing and circulation become free. The patient feels lighter, breathes and walks

easier. Instead of having to use the body vitality for digestive work, it can be directed toward neutralization of poisons. This demonstrable improvement of the patient is also reflected in his general outlook and cheerfulness.

... The main feature in the treatment was fasting from twenty-five to thirty days, combined with air and sunbaths

In the history of medicine, many fasts prescribed by physicians are recorded. Hippocrates suggested fasts up to seven days and stated: "Hunger reacts in the nature of man with great power and can be considered the means that leads to recovery from disease."

But by the nineteenth century, fasting came to be thought of as a thing of the past. The sick had to be well nourished. Even fever patients had to be substantially fed. The benefits of fasting were virtually forgotten.

But now the medically supervised fast is really coming into its own—with solid evidence from many doctors and researches as to its therapeutic value.

Dr. Maxwell O. Garten, a great believer in fasting, and under whose supervision I experienced my first fast, says:

At the beginning of the fast, the body draws first upon its stored glycogen (muscle sugar). After all reserves have been used up, certain enzymes in the bloodstream receive special attention and become intensified in their ability to dissolve hardened infusions. Since these fluids can reach each and every cell, they soon exert their liquefying action. The cholesterol attached to the inside wall of the vessels, like the scale in the water kettle, begins to melt and is carried away to be used by the body as food. The same principles apply to other deposits, such as uric acid, calcium carbonate and chlorine.

Under the emergency of food withholding, the body economy is enabled to not only "turn back the clock" and reshuffle the chemistry of the invaded blockade deposits, but also to revaluate the consistency of the tissues and organs themselves. ... It can be said that during the fast, the body lives on its own reserves.

During World War II the problem of survival without food became acute. However, scientific experiments proved that American soldiers could live sixty days without food. After that the body gradually begins to starve. Through animal experiments it has been found that the point at which death from starvation begins is proportional to the cube root of the body weight. For example, a mouse weighing 18.0 grams dies after six days without food. A dog weighing 20 pounds dies in sixty days. It has been said that man can live from ninety to one hundred days without food, if he were kept under proper conditions of warmth, rest, fresh air, water and emotional poise.

Upton Sinclair, who was a devoted follower of fasting, said in an article in *Cosmopolitan*:

> Can you form any image of what would be your feeling if every organ in your body were functioning perfectly? ... It is simply that for ten years I have been studying the ill health of myself and of the men and women around me and I have found the cause and remedy. I have not only found good health but perfect health; I have found a new state of being, a new potentiality of life; a sense of lightness and cleanness and joyfulness such as I did not know could exist in the human body.

To quote Mr. Sinclair from another article also from the *Cosmopolitan* magazine:

> There are two dangers to be feared in fasting. The first is that of fear. I do not say this as a jest. The faster should not have about him terrified aunts and cousins who will tell him that he looks like a corpse, that his pulse is below forty and that his heart may stop beating in the night. I took a fast of three days out in California, on the third day I walked 15 miles, off and on, and, except that I was restless, I never felt better; and then in the evening I came home and read about the Messina earthquake, and how the relief ships arrived, and the wretched survivors crowded down to the water's edge and tore each other like wild beasts in their rage of hunger. The paper set forth, in horrified language, that some of them had been 72 hours without food. I, as I read, had also been 72 hours without food, and the difference was simply that they thought they were starving.

The mind during the fast is of utmost importance. There is no question that fasting is an unusual experience for most people.

There is likely to be a feeling of anxiety and uncertainty. Such insecure feelings may be intensified by well-meaning but ignorant members of the home. The Bible says, "A man's foes shall be they of his own household."

A *Reader's Digest* article* in the November 1962 issue contained the following statement regarding fasts:

> Modern medical science is turning to an ancient practice—total fasting—and finding that when properly supervised it is safe, painless and effective. . . . Dramatic results, painlessly achieved, give the overweight person fresh confidence and help to lead him back to a balanced diet of caloric content sufficient to meet his needs.
>
> Fasting for other than weight-reduction purposes is an honored and ancient practice. The Old and New testaments mention it 74 times. Christ fasted forty days and forty nights. In Islam there is the universally observed thirty-day, sunup-to-sundown fast of Ramadan, and Buddhists find fasting appropriate to their way of contemplation and asceticism.
>
> Perhaps the most carefully observed forbearance from eating was that of A. Levanzin, a lawyer and publisher in Malta, who believed that fasting had cured him, his wife and their two children of serious illnesses. In 1912 he came to the Carnegie Institution in Boston and submitted himself to a 31-day study. Levanzin, who weighed 134, lived under the closest scrutiny day and night, existing on nothing but distilled water. A retinue of specialists made daily tests and observations of his physical condition, his subjective impressions and mental attitude.
>
> As he himself had predicted, Levanzin had no sensation of hunger, and no desire for food. He experienced no abdominal pain nor discomfort. On the 11th day, he was conscious of muscular fatigue, but on the 14th day he ran down a flight of stairs without difficulty. His memory, tested daily, was as good at the end as at the beginning.

There are certain rules to observe during the fast and therefore *it is absolutely essential to do it under the supervision of a doctor.* Complete fasts should never be undertaken without close and qualified supervision.

When Gandhi was submitting to one of his widely publicized

* *A Swift, Sure Way to Take Off Weight,* by Blake Clark.

tasts, he was attended by a physician who proclaimed him to be as healthy as a man of forty despite his age of sixty-four.

This book could be filled with similar examples, but again, I want to stress that fasting can only be done safely under professional supervision.

Climate, nutrition, earthbound simplicity, emotional balance— undoubtedly all these factors contribute to the exceptional physical condition of the people of Hunza.

But the seasonal scarcity of food to which they are subjected each spring is one health-giving factor that has been largely overlooked. The high elevation and restricted farming land limit their production of foodstuffs to dangerously low levels for existing needs. Come early spring and last year's harvest has been consumed. A few potatoes may be left, perhaps, and a little grain or some dried apricots. Frequently, however, there is very little left of any edibles, and the people simply have to wait for the new crop of fruit, berries, grains and vegetables. They turn thin and scrawny, but they do not forget how to smile. They go on with their work with a friendly attitude and faith that soon they will have plenty of food.

The enforced fast undoubtedly has its rejuvenating effect. The cells, tissue and organs, deprived of all unused and precipitated blockade materials, are ready to be replenished anew.

This physical *rebirth*, as it were, might well be a major factor in the physical superiority of the Hunzakuts. And it is more than likely that their seasonal fasts tend to keep them humble, friendly, helpful and devotional.

13.

Exercises
for Health
and Longevity

In addition to proper nutrition and a strong spiritual outlook, there is still another vital factor in the Hunza recipe for good health. That factor is exercise. In Hunza, the people are almost constantly exercising as they go about their work in the mountain fields, constantly keeping their muscles well toned.

But what about the city dwellers of the Western world who journey through life in a car or train? If we are to retain our health we, too, must have sufficient exercise.

There is no excuse for not having daily exercise. The easiest, the most readily available and the most inexpensive exercise is walking. Plain, honest, everyday putting-the-right-foot-in-front-of-the-left-foot walking. I realize that many people regard walking simply as a last resort, but it can be fun if you know how to make it so. If you are not fortunate enough to be within easy access of hillsides or ocean views, try to see how many new things you can discover while taking a turn around the block, or several blocks. You will probably be amazed at the number of things which have previously escaped your notice.

(I read somewhere that Henry Ford refused to have an elevator in his huge home; he always walked up the stairs no matter how many flights were ahead of him.)

The medical profession has accepted the value of walking as an essential part of our health program. In fact, after a serious operation today, a patient is forced to get out of bed and walk the very next day. Recently I visited a friend of mine in a San Diego hospital who had undergone a major operation. On the second day he was out of bed and walking in spite of all the pain and discomfort. A week later he was sent home. Doctors urge patients to move around so that their leg muscles will not become idle and blood clots will not form easily.

The Hunzakut people are the best proof that walking is beneficial. They walk for miles every day, since they have no vehicles. Their fields are usually quite far from their homes and as a rule located on hillsides. Then men also travel from village to village, 10 to 15 miles each way, and some of them walk to Gilgit, 68 miles from Baltit, their capital. This is done in one stretch, and if they return home in the daytime, they go about their work as though they have just come from taking a nap.

No matter what your business, it is imperative that you designate at least a few minutes each day to exercise, for exercise is a health- and beauty-builder and will keep your body youthful.

Exercise keeps you physically and mentally alive, for only through exercise can the necessary flow of oxygen be brought into your blood to keep your system functioning normally. With a healthy circulation of blood, the waste materials can be removed from the body and will not be encouraged to linger on to cause fatigue.

Fat will seldom leave its deposits in an active body. Aside from those individuals with glandular ills, no active person need be fat or flabby. In Hunza, where hiking is a daily necessity, you will not find a single overweight person.

The greatest percentage of our bodies is composed of muscle. And when those muscles are not properly exercised they not only become flabby but they slowly quicken the process of body deterioration. Lack of exercise brings on old age.

How often we mistakenly assume that because we are becoming advanced in years that we must, if we intend to live a long life, cut down the extent of our physical exercise. We fail to realize that by limiting our activities, we are doing exactly the opposite of what we set out to do—indeed we may be cutting our life expectancy in half!

I read an amusing article, "Walking," by J. I. Rodale, Editor of *Prevention* magazine, in April 1962 issue: . . . "An anecdote involving Dr. Thomas Sydenham, known as the father of English medicine who lived in the 1600's. It seems he had a patient with the gout but all his remedies proved ineffective. So he sent him to see a certain doctor about a hundred miles from London, who he said was the world's greatest authority on the gout.

"The patient soon found that there was no stagecoach that went to this town so he had to ride a hundred miles on horseback to see the doctor. But when he got there, nobody had ever heard of the doctor he had come to see. So he rode the hundred miles back to London, called on Dr. Sydenham, and asked him, 'On what kind of wild-goose chase did you send me?' The doctor replied by asking him 'How's your gout?' 'What gout,' replied the patient. The physical action of 200 miles on a horse's back, the perspiration it produced, the oxygen it sent into all the obscure parts of his body, the hormones that his glands made, all contributed to clearing up the symptoms of the man's gout."

If, like the Hunzakuts, you exercise daily, your muscles will remain active, young and healthy as long as you live.

There are many varied forms of beneficial exercises, and many books have been written on physical fitness and exercises. I choose the yoga technique. Yoga exercises were devised about six thousand years ago, originally created by the great teachers of the ancient East.

I have studied yoga for many years under the guidance of Indra Devi, yoga teacher and author of many books on the subject. She is the only Occidental woman ever to teach yoga in India. She lived there for many years and mastered the techniques to perfection.

The word "yoga" is derived from the Sanskrit root *yug*, which means to unite, or bring together. It is a practical system of thought and methods leading to the supreme union—the union between God and the individual soul.

In our Western world the concept of yoga has been confused with magic and the supernatural. Recently, though, it has been accepted as an excellent form of physical exercise and has become popular among many people.

The definition of "yoga" given by Patanjali, the great father of the yoga system, is simple and clear: yoga gives us power to control mental waves—such as sadness, depression, anger and unrest. These waves arise from any kind of mental disturbance. The person who learns to control these waves has conquered life itself.

Yoga is a pure psychology of thought, mind and culture. It teaches a man how he can master himself, how he can gain control over his body and his undesirable habits. Whether people live in the East or in the West, a man who has attained the results of the yoga system through concentration, self-control and tranquility arrives at a state of consciousness where he transcends the limits of the flesh. Anyone can adopt this technique and practice it to great satisfaction.

The yoga system is divided into many parts. The first step begins with the body. You must prove that you can bring your hands, your feet and every limb of your body, your eyes, your ears and all your senses to order and coordination. You must learn to concentrate and sit still without a feeling of strain or nervous confusion.

Can everyone practice yoga? Of course! There is no need to go through intricate ways of breathing, or postures that intimidate so many people or complicated mental processes.

Hatha yoga, known as the first steps of yoga, teaches a simple method of correct, deep rhythmic breathing, then relaxation, and also teaches you to improve your posture, voice, eyesight and eating habits. It means that everything we do—such as eating, drinking, sleeping, working—has a significance, and if we learn how to do these things properly, with moderation and tranquility, we shall be practicing what yoga teaches. Simple, isn't it? Once and for all, let us understand that yoga is not a religion—it is a way of life. We cannot lead a disorderly life and expect to have mental coordination and a body which enjoys health. Our thoughts and actions must become harmonious.

It is not a question of spending a great deal of time to practice yoga. In our busy world it wouldn't be practical, so a period of fifteen to twenty minutes daily set aside for our mental and physical training will bring great benefits. These exercises stimulate every part of the body, including muscles, nerves and glands—thus regulating our entire system. As a result, a stout person will lose his fat, whereas an underweight person gains missing pounds. The various postures maintain the body in proper weight and shape.

Most of us have been taught from childhood to breathe the wrong way, through unnatural expansion of the chest. It is essential to learn to breathe correctly. Thousands of years ago the yogis recognized the amazing results of regulating breathing for maintaining health. They practically made religious ceremonies out of deep rhythmic breathing exercises combined with physical postures. According to their theories, postures without the breathing exercises did not produce the same results.

The yogis planned the exercises for everyone as a daily routine. Breath, or *prana*, is the living force. Without prana there is no life, for prana is the soul of all force and all energy, and the human organism absorbs prana from the air through the process of breathing. Of course, we have to breathe to live. We can live without food for days, but we cannot live without air.

Through controlled, rhythmic deep breathing the intake of prana is increased and you are able to store up a substantial quantity of reserve in your brain and nerve centers to be used in an emergency.

People who practice deep breathing possess greater vitality, endurance, and better control of the mind. By regular practice of breathing you store up that additional oxygen.

Recently I learned that yoga had been practiced by the Hunza people of many generations ago. And it is obvious that they continue to practice what their forefathers had learned, even though they are not aware of it.

The Hunza people use the correct technique of deep breathing. If they did not, they would have difficulty in doing such strenuous work in high altitude. Moreover, they walk gracefully, carrying their bodies with a sense of how each part should be used. They are slender and well proportioned. They eat simple foods, and a little at a time.

All the basic principles of yoga technique are practiced by these people who live on the world's rooftop.

DEEP-BREATHING TECHNIQUE

Deep rhythmic breathing is the first lesson of yoga.

1. Deep breathing should always be done in a well-ventilated room or at an open window, weather permitting.
2. Wear comfortable clothes—no girdle or brassière.

3. Do it on an empty stomach.

4. The ideal position is sitting crossed-legged on a rug or blanket on the floor.

5. It also can be done sitting in a comfortable chair, placing your hands on your knees or standing up. If a person is bedridden, it can be done lying flat on the bed.

6. Relax your whole body and keep the spine straight.

7. We determine our rhythm by listening and counting our own pulse. First count aloud, one-two-three-four; one-two-three-four; then count mentally, and when you are sure of your own rhythm you are ready to begin the exercises.

8. Now count mentally four pulsebeats while inhaling and four pulsebeats while exhaling. The breath should flow smoothly and not staccatolike when you do the counting. You have just taken one complete breathing exercise. Repeat the same routine four times. In the beginning do not do it more than four times. After a week you can add one exercise weekly until you reach sixty a day. However do not do them in one session. Divide them into two or three sessions daily: in the morning, during the day and in the evening before going to sleep. However, always remember to follow the instructions given above. Always inhale four in and four out.

9. Breathe by slightly contracting the throat (this will partly close the epiglottis) and slowly inhale a breath, keeping the mouth shut. There will be a slight hissing sound coming from the back of the throat, which will be the indication that you are doing the breathing correctly.

10. Never raise your chest while inhaling. Let your rib cage expand on both sides. Then slowly exhale with the same hissing sound while contracting the rib cage and slightly pulling in your stomach.

11. Once you learn the correct technique of deep breathing and do these exercises regularly you will feel a definite improvement in your general well-being.

12. However, you must remember that this way of breathing is an exercise and you should not attempt it all the time.

13. Children should learn the same technique so that they do not have difficulties later. It is said that babies and savages are the only ones who know the technique of instinctive breathing. When children get in touch with modern civilization, they lose the ability to

breathe naturally. Therefore, correct rhythmic breathing should be taught in kindergarten.

14. When inhaling, concentrate on the intake of fresh air filled with oxygen, and visualize it entering into your lungs. In case you have a weak spot in your body which occasionally causes discomfort or pain, try to direct your intake of prana into that particular spot. Remember, when you inhale you get fresh air into your system, and exhaling you get carbon dioxide (poison) out of your system.

The yogis maintain that proper breathing attunes one to the "rhythm of the universe." According to their thinking, everything that lives and moves has a rhythm, and we can live and function harmoniously as long as we keep to our individual rhythm. Anyone can do the rhythmic deep-breathing exercises to control his well-being.

YOGA EXERCISES

A few basic exercises should be practiced daily.

1. Wear comfortable clothes such as a bathing suit or leotards.

2. Exercise on a surface that is neither too hard nor too soft.

3. Choose a corner of the floor that has adequate room for you to move around.

4. The morning hours are usually recommended. It helps to start the day with additional vigor.

5. Exercise always on an empty stomach and not longer than one hour at a time.

6. Rest frequently in between the various postures so that you never tire yourself during practice. These particular postures should give you a feeling of complete comfort and relaxation, otherwise no benefit will be derived from them.

7. Every exercise should be coupled with deep breathing. Inhale through the nostrils with mouth closed.

8. Of course, you should check out any exercise program with your doctor if you are not in perfect health.

STRETCHING

Do the stretching while you are still in bed. Flat on your back, begin to stretch one leg counting slowly, one-two-three up to ten to begin with, continuing to stretch the leg forward. Then bring it back and repeat the same with the other leg. Add one more count every day until you can count to thirty. Stretching is a wonderful way to build up control of your muscles.

Get out of bed, stand straight in front of an open window and do a few breathing exercises. Then stretch with your arms high above your head. Then swing slightly to the left and right a few times. Repeat this ten times, inhaling as you stretch and exhaling as you swing.

Stretch your hands high over your head and slowly begin to swing your arms from left to right, lowering them inch-by-inch, relaxing your whole body until you reach the floor with the tips of your fingers. Then start swinging back in the same manner, with the same rhythm, bringing your arms inch-by-inch up to the original position. Stretch the arms and then let them go, returning them to your sides. Repeat this twice.

THE STOMACH LIFT

Stand erect, keeping your feet apart. Inhale deeply, exhale and, without taking a new breath, pull your abdomen in so that it becomes hollow. Now slightly bend your knees forward, place hands on thighs, inclining the body a little forward. Do not breathe at all while in action. Now pull the stomach in and out, repeating it as long as you can hold your breath without feeling tired. Return to the original posture and repeat the exercise ten times. This posture is considered an excellent antidote for a flabby stomach, as it strengthens abdominal muscles. It also helps to reduce constipation, indigestion, etc.

ROCKING EXERCISE

Sit on the floor and raise both knees, keeping feet on the ground, hands under the knees. Bend forward and start rocking back and forth about ten times without stopping and without straightening the spine. Do this exercise whenever you feel tired or have been sitting too long. After watching television for any length of time, get on the floor and rock for a few times to limber up. In case your spine is sensitive, use an extra padding on the floor.

THE LOTUS POSTURE

This exercise has been adopted for meditation. The ancient philosophers and teachers who designed the yoga techniques found it most suitable for concentration.

1. Sit down on the floor, crossing your legs, placing each heel on the opposite thigh. In the beginning it is not necessary to attempt sitting in the proper lotus posture. It can be accomplished simply by sitting criss-crossed, tailor fashion, keeping your knees on the floor. Try to sit straight.

2. Clasp your hands behind your back, take a deep breath and then, exhaling, bend forward till your forehead touches the floor. Remain motionless for a few seconds, then return slowly to the original position. Do not force reaching the floor at the start. This will come when your whole body becomes supple and strong.

3. Do not strain or force any part of your body.

4. Remaining in the same position with your hands clasped, sit straight, take a deep breath and, while exhaling, bend to the right until your forehead reaches your knee, then slowly return to the original position. Repeat the same to the left side. Repeat all three postures four times.

Neck Exercises

Sit in the same position as for the lotus posture or on the chair if you cannot get down on the floor. Keep your spine straight and eyes closed.

1. Throw the head back, then forward.

2. Turn the head to the right with a jerk, then to the left with a jerk.

3. The head sideways to the right, then sideways to the left.

4. Rotate the head clockwise and counterclockwise.

Repeat each exercise ten times.

Eye Exercises

Remain sitting in the same position, open your eyes and do the following exercises without moving your head.

1. Look up to the ceiling and then down to the floor.

2. Move your eyes to the right, then to the left.

3. Then to the right corner up, to the left corner down.

4. Repeat, moving your eyes to the left corner up, and then right corner down.

5. Roll eyes clockwise and counterclockwise.

Repeat each one six times and blink several times after each exercise. Close your eyes gently after each exercise.

6. Then do the *shifting of the eyes*. Choose an object close to the eyes, then shift them to an object in the far distance. Repeat this a few times, then blink your eyes to let them rest for a while.

PALMING OF THE EYES

Cover both eyes with cupped hands. Rest the heel of palms on cheekbones without pressing them, fingers crossed over forehead. Don't touch the eyeballs with the palms. Close your eyes lightly, without strain. Try to make sure that all light is excluded. To get good results from this exercise, your head should not be bent forward. The back of your neck and spine must be comfortable and absolutely straight so that there is no strain on your nerves or muscles. Place your elbows on a pillow to elevate the position of your elbow. The best place to rest the elbows is on a low table. Palming is an excellent method for relaxation and to relieve common strain. Everyone should practice it a few times a day. You can do it right at your desk at work. Palming is particularly beneficial to persons whose work requires a great deal of reading or figure work. There are thousands of nerve centers embedded within the palm of the hand, and it is quite likely that the old masters of the East practiced palming to increase magnetic forces. Therefore it is possible that more than sight can be enhanced by palming. Palm for about ten minutes at a time. Do your deep breathing during the palming. After a while you will feel wonderfully rested.

SWINGING

Stand with your feet apart, hands loosely at your sides. Relax and start swinging your whole body from left to right, simultaneously lifting the heel of the opposite foot. The head and eyes and arms should follow the motion of the body with perfect ease and without any strain. This exercise relaxes the eyes, the spine and the back, and your mind will relax, too, with the rhythm of your swinging.

SUNNING

It is good to sun your eyes but do not expose both eyes at the same time. One eye must be covered with your palm while the other eye is exposed to the sun. Rotate the eyes, exposing each one to the sun for a few seconds only. Never stare at the sun with both eyes.

AN EXERCISE FOR LEGS, THIGHS AND OTHER JOINTS

1. Sit on chair, keeping your spine straight and body completely relaxed.

2. Raise right leg up and down, then left leg. Repeat the same.

3. Raise both legs up and down.

4. Then raise both legs and criss-cross them, repeating same a few times. Increase the amount of every variation daily but do not overdo any one of them.

THE COBRA POSTURE

1. Lie face down on floor and place your palms on either side of your chest.

2. Keep your legs together, toes pointed.

3. Inhale a deep breath and while doing so raise the upper part of your body, leaning on your hands and arching the back.

4. Throw your head back, holding your breath. Remain for a few seconds.

5. Slowly return to the original position while exhaling.

TO STRENGTHEN BACK MUSCLES

Lie on the floor face down. Bring your hands together over your back. Take a deep breath and raise your legs and head as high as possible while holding your breath. Return to the original position, exhaling slowly. Repeat a few times, then relax in the same position, lying flat on your stomach.

SLANT BOARD

Certain exercises, especially for relaxation, can be done on a *slant board*. It is a simple board which is raised about 15 inches at one end. If you lie in a position with your head lower than your feet, the blood has the opportunity to flow freely to your head, chin, throat and cheeks, which increases the blood circulation and in turn increases the functioning of your mind. By relaxing your feet, the tension of the foot muscles is released. Other benefits to be derived from this position are added circulation to scalp and facial muscles.

Gayelord Hauser calls it "the magic yoga slant." He says anyone can lie on the slant board regardless of age.

The headstand is practiced a great deal by the yoga students and considered one of the most beneficial postures because of the increased blood supply to the head. However, it must be done under supervision. The slant board would serve the same purpose to some extent, and there is no danger whatever involved in doing it by yourself. And while on the slant board you can do your breathing and relaxation exercises.

Gayelord Hauser recommends a "stomach lift" to be done on the slant board. Lying relaxed, draw in your stomach as you count one. Draw your stomach in and up, further, on the count of two. On the count of three, draw it in close to your spine, which is pressing flat against the board. Try to hold this position to the count of ten. Then relax. This is an excellent exercise to firm up the abdominal muscles and keep the waistline trim and youthful.

Most beauty and health farms use slant boards as part of their daily routine.

Everyone should have a slant board next to his bed. A friend of mine wakes up early in the morning and slides onto her slant board and continues her sleep until it is time to get up. She claims it relaxes her for the rest of the day.

You can buy a slant board very inexpensively at your health-food store.

After a series of exercises a few minutes should be devoted to relaxation.

Lie flat on your back with hands on both sides and eyes closed. Relax all muscles from top to toe. Roll to one side and relax completely in this position for a minute, then roll to the other side and remain relaxed in the same manner. Return to your original position (flat on your back) and begin relaxing your head, facial muscles, neck, shoulders, arms, forearms, elbows and fingers, then relax your thighs, legs, ankles, toes and knees.

Draw a picture of beauty and peace in your mind, seeing yourself amidst beautiful surroundings. Think of the magnificent valley of Hunza. Keep completely relaxed. Remain in this position for a few minutes. Then slowly start stretching: stretch your arms, your feet, roll to one side, then to the other . . . open your eyes and slowly get up. You should feel that life is pulsating through your body. You should experience mental peace and new vigor. Try to do this exercise every day.

Anyone who learns the technique of relaxation can do it any-where. You can put your mind at ease by snapping a finger, and

become unaware of the noise around you. Being able to relax even
for a few minutes will supply the body with new energy. Those
who practice this daily will soon discover how to conserve their
physical and mental energy and utilize it to their best advantage.
The Hunzakuts, with their seemingly endless energy, have proved
this to be a fact.

We blame the automobile for slowing down our motions. This
does not have to be. While driving you can do your breathing exercises. *Don't* do them in a crowded city filled with gasoline odors!

Do your neck exercises in the bathroom.

Do your stretching while still in bed.

You will find time for everything if you once make up your
mind that this is what you want. So be determined and practice
your exercises daily.

Dr. Paul Dudley White, in a pamphlet entitled *Exercise Is Good
Preventive Medicine*, stresses the importance of exercises for general health:

> Exercise is important for everybody, whether they've been
> sick or not. Of course, a person with an acute illness, whether
> it's from heart disease or pneumonia or any other kind of
> illness, has to be treated for that immediate disease. But after
> recovery, graded exercise can favor the progress of conva-
> lescence and rehabilitation. There are immediate physical
> benefits of exercise on the circulation of the blood. Good
> muscle tone in the arms and particularly in the legs, resulting
> from regular exercise, maintains an improved circulation of
> blood in the veins. . . . It matters little, if at all, what type of
> exercise it is, provided it suits the strength and liking of the
> individual concerned. It is well to establish a regular habit
> and to maintain it through thick and thin. One should regard
> it just as essential to good health as eating, sleeping and
> working.

Be aware of your body, your posture, your face and your
beauty. Try to walk gracefully, keep your body straight, pulling
the stomach in. Sit straight when you type and when you write
letters. Stretch gracefully.

Swimming is another splendid form of exercise. There is a community swimming pool in every village in Hunza, and the people
swim in this very cold water of melted snow. They believe that the
body should get used to various temperatures.

Remember, health comes above everything else. A longer, healthier life will be your reward.

THE SCIENCE OF SOUNDS

Singing is gradually disappearing from our modern way of living. It is so much easier to turn on the radio or look at television. But the Hunzakuts enjoy singing and accompany most of their work with cheerful songs. In school the boys have one solid hour of singing, then an hour of exercising. The rest of the time is devoted to studying.

Why not start singing in the bathroom again?

The yogis have devised special sounds called *mantras*, which are based on certain vowel combinations. The mantras are chanted in a specific manner so as to produce a vibrating effect on our entire system, the nerves, glands and brain.

The Hunzakuts chant morning and evening during their prayers. They practice the sound vibrations, unaware of the excellent effect it has on their health. It is simply a tradition which has been passed down for centuries.

My day starts with mantras, and I go through the routine of a few vowels ... *E* ... *A* ... *O* ... *U* ..., which are done in the following manner:

Inhale first, then without exhaling sound a strong and piercing *eeeeeeeeeeeeeeeee*, holding your mouth as in a smile. The sound should be even and kept on the same pitch. Stop before you are completely out of breath. Rest and repeat the vowel again. Follow the same routine with the other vowels, using each separately.

Don't read this book and say, "Yes, I must start exercising. I think I shall start tomorrow." Tomorrow may never come if you don't start today. Don't *think* about exercising—*do* it! Like the Hunzakuts—make it an integral part of your life, and make your own Shangri-la.

14.

Soil and Survival

We are told to eat a little of this and a little of that ... foods that contain Vitamins A, B, C and so on, but what do the Hunzakuts know about this alphabet of nutritive values? Their nutrition comes from the foods they grow in their fields and have grown in the same soil for centuries.

Thus the question arises: Is the circle of health complete? Are the crops, the animals and the vegetation as healthy as the people of Hunza themselves?

Plant life is by its nature less mobile than man's. Movement is only by winged or carried seed, and is limited. Therefore one would expect that the making of plant life in man's image would have a far more serious effect on plants than on man. Indeed I sometimes marvel that plants have survived some of the great disturbances to which they have been subjected. It argues much for the scientific skill of man that he should have been able to bring about so many changes at all. But nevertheless, nature hits back, and she hits back with disease.

The Mir has said to me, "If you take a loan from the bank, you have to pay it back. If you don't pay it back you won't get any more money." The same applies to the soil—what you take out of it you must put back.

The Hunzakuts are fortunate. They enrich their soil with rich mineral water and they enrich it with natural fertilizer prepared by man from the things he has taken out of the soil. They carefully collect the cattle manure, all vegetable parts which are not for animal or human consumption, fallen leaves and ashes from their fires. Everything is mixed together and made into compost. Then some alkaline earth is spread over the fields during irrigation. This enriched soil produces the rich plants which serve as food and bring all the essential goodness needed to build healthy bodies.

The Hunzakuts garden their fields the way we do our gardens— it is a constant and never-ending job. Everything that once had life is brought back to life by loving hands. This form of culture has produced excellent food, and plant disease is insignificant.

It is possible that by full repayment to the soil we alone get a full return. We have worked our soil—raided our soil—without replenishing it. And only when the soil sickens do we doctor it with artificial tonics of nitrogen, calcium and phosphorus which we originally took out and forgot to return.

We have to look back to the period of our agriculture when our soil and our animals were healthy; to the time when men were bestowed with the gift of health through plants and fruits.

Sir Albert Howard, an English scientist stationed in Asia, made a study of the relationship of plant, soil and animal. He writes in *The Role of Insects and Fungi in Agriculture*:*

> I was able to study the reaction of well-fed animals to epidemic diseases, such as rinderpest, foot-and-mouth disease, septicaemia, and so forth, which frequently devastated the countryside. None of my animals was segregated; none was inoculated; they frequently came in contact with diseased stock. No case of infectious disease occurred. The reward of well-nourished protoplasm was a very high degree of disease resistance, which might even be described as immunity.

Howard's two principal conclusions in this paper are highly important and most timely.

> 1. Insects and fungi are not the real cause of plant diseases, and only attack unsuitable varieties of crops improperly grown. Their true role in agriculture is that of censors for pointing out the crops which are imperfectly nourished.

* *The Empire Cotton Growing Review*, Vol. XIII.

Disease resistance seems to be the natural reward of health and well-nourished protoplasm. The first step is to make the soil live by seeing that the supply of humus is maintained.

2. The policy of protecting crops from pests by means of sprays, powders, and so forth is thoroughly unscientific and radically unsound; even when successful, this procedure merely preserves materials hardly worth saving. The annihilation or avoidance of a pest involves the destruction of the real problem; such methods constitute no scientific solution of the trouble, but are mere evasions.

. . . . . .
. . . . . .

And here is tiny Hunza, where there is practically no human disease, no animal disease and no plant disease. But then, they don't contaminate their plants and their soil. Their food is pure, fresh and healthful. All the things that our teachers and nutritionists recommend that we do, the Hunzakuts have done for centuries.

Commercial fertilizers are usually made up of nitrogen, phosphoric acid and potash in varying proportions. The traditional assumption has been that all other mineral elements are always in the soil in sufficient quantities to meet the needs of growing crops. This assumption is gratuitous and without foundation in fact. All these elements and ingredients may be in the soil and bountiful crops be produced and yet there may be a decided lack of the minor but essential things that go into food for man. There are soils so peculiarly constituted that they need minerals that are in no sense of the word fertilizers. Some need copper and sulphate, some manganese, some lime, etc. Doctoring soils is as yet purely empirical, experimental. It is not an established science.

Quantity production can be had by both compost and commercial-fertilizer methods. But is one as good as the other? And, more important, is one as beneficial to man and soil alike as the other?

Experts argue that soil treated with the compost method will remain in perfect condition, while soil "enriched" with commercial fertilizers will soon become barren and deserted by those creatures which inhabit it and make it fertile.

The soil, in order to remain fertile, must maintain a balanced amount of mineral elements. But from where do these elements come? From the near-microscopic inhabitants of the earth? Or can they be successfully added to the soil by means of artificial restoration? But then again, as in the case of modern milling processes, why must we remove the vital source of mineral energy to begin with? Doesn't this only result in twice as much work? And are the minerals which are "replanted" into the soil as efficient as those which time and constant use of the soil has taken away?

What is it that constitutes a truly fertile soil? Is it a soil which can produce a bountiful yield of produce? No. Fertile soil is soil which can yield quality produce as well as great quantities of produce. Physicians have proved that a man can consume three large meals each day and still die of malnutrition. Tests have shown that malnutrition can be induced by foods grown in fields fertilized with commercial fertilizer.

The relation of soil and health is a vital part of the study of nutrition. The problem is wrapped up and deposited before us, and we must examine it. It has recently been discovered that human health is closely related to the plant-food elements in the soil from which the food is obtained. The only way to get the elements vital to our survival is to consume them. But are the foods we eat supplying us with these imperative elements? They cannot if the soil which has grown them is itself suffering from lack of these elements. So, we must think about replenishing the land which has given us sustenance.

Shall we use commercial fertilizers? Or shall we eat only foods which are grown in compost gardens? Unfortunately, it is not that simple. Neither method is perfect. Perhaps the answer lies in the joint usage of both. A compost rich in natural materials is useless unless it contains a like amount of raw minerals. On the other hand, a chemically proficient fertilizer which is rich in minerals, is useless without humus or decayed vegetation or potash and nitrogen.

It is a known fact that the human body must contain various vitamins and mineral elements in varying proportions. These vitamins and minerals are most effective when introduced into the system through the workings of the digestive tract. Since plants get their food essentially from the soil, it stands to reason that the plant can only contain those elements which the soil can give forth. A balanced ration for human beings is dependent on a balanced ration for plants and soil.

As we all know, long life is dependent on health, health is dependent on food and food is in turn dependent on the soil. Even meat comes mostly from land animals which get their food from plants.

Plants will grow in compost soil with very few minerals. They will also grow with no compost at all, either in soil or in mineralized water. Hydroponics, the cultivation of plants by placing the roots in liquid nutrient solutions rather than in soil, have proved this. So the claim that compost soil is absolutely necessary for the development of healthy plants is false. Obviously the key to healthy plant production is giving the plants the proper amount of minerals. Plants will grow in soil. They will grow in mineralized water. And plants set in gravel and nourished with enriched water will flourish splendidly, as hydroponics has shown. Yet, whether grown in soil or in water, the amount of minerals must be rationed properly. Therein lies another problem. What is the proper amount of minerals necessary to fully nourish a plant? What minerals are essential?

Commercial fertilizer proves an expensive proposition when used on large acreages. Therefore, at least for the present, the only practical alternative is the one farmers and agricultural experts have reached. Crops are rotated, soil-improving crops are favored by the farmer and humus is produced in the soil where extensive and continuous farming is practiced.

This does not, however, guarantee that the crops produced will be rich in minerals. It cannot guarantee even that the soil will be rich in minerals. All it can promise is that the soil will be adequate.

. . . . . .
. . . . . .

It is an accepted fact among biochemists that the human body needs many different minerals if it is to function properly. Since no one wants to be sick or feel left out of things or always be in the direct path to those innumerable ailments which "flesh is heir to," we must wake up to the fact that we truly are what we eat. We must begin to put to work the preventive agencies and, by giving our soil and foods a clean bill of health, insure our own good health.

Dr. H. D. Brown, professor of horticulture, and Chester B. Hutchinson in their book *Vegetable Science*, write: "The farmers of the United States have dissipated the native fertility of the soils more rapidly than have the farmers of any other country. . . . They have removed (in crops) the minerals from the land. . . ."

Arnold P. Yerkes writes in his *Soil: A Foundation of Health*:

> You may wonder why certain elements are missing in our farm soils today if they were once present. You will doubtless also wonder why something has not been done to replace these depleted elements if they are so important in maintaining the health of plants, animals, and human beings.
>
> . . . . . .
>
> The virgin soils in the United States, when it was first settled by white men, were not all alike so far as mineral content and other characteristics were concerned. But most of them probably contained adequate quantities of most of the minerals listed as being required for human health.
>
> . . . . . .
>
> The story of how some of these minerals were removed from the soils to a point where their lack causes disease and insect-ridden plants, sickly animals, and menaces to the health of the entire population, must be limited to a few words.
>
> For many generations crop and animals have been grown on our farm lands and shipped to the cities. With them, at first, went the minerals which nature intended they should contain. Each year's crop contained only small quantities of these "minor" elements, but in the one or two hundred years that our better soils have been farmed, some of these important "minor" elements have been depleted. Erosion and leaching have lent a strong hand in this process in many areas.
>
> The minerals shipped to the cities never returned to the soil of the farms from which they were hauled, instead, they went back to the sea as sewage or landed in inaccessible spots such as garbage dumps or ash heaps. While animal bones

were ground into meal by the farms where it was needed to produce health-giving food.

It is a fair question to ask why no one protested against this continued removal of these vital minerals from the farm lands without any effort being made to replace them. The answer is that a few people did realize what was going on and tried to warn the public. They protested against the waste of minerals through our methods of disposing of garbage and sewage. For the most part they were voices crying in the wilderness.

. . . . . .

Plants do perform some near-miracles, but they simply can't extract from a soil minerals which are no longer there. They will always do their best to grow and produce seed to perpetuate their species, but when the soil is exhausted of certain minerals the plant cannot enjoy real health. We know that some so-called plant "diseases" are really the effects of the absence of certain minerals. It seems probable that others may be found to be in the same class.

Some people think all such "diseases" are just the effects of deficiencies. They even claim insect damage is often due to the unhealthy condition caused by such deficiencies . . . that healthy plants are not so appetizing to bugs and that they can better withstand their attacks.

Others scoff at such beliefs, and much time and printer's ink have been wasted in arguing the case. We should not tolerate arguments and "opinions" on such important matters in this day and age, when the facilities are available to obtain the facts.

You may wonder why certain elements are missing in our farm soils today if they were once present. You will doubtless also wonder why something has not been done to replace these depleted elements if they are so important in maintaining the health of plants, animals, and human beings.

Exactly what is soil and why, specifically, is it so vital to human health?

Geologically speaking, soils are made up of ground and pulverized minerals that hold intact all soluble plant-food elements which need moisture, air and sunshine to cause seed to germinate and, ultimately, to produce growth. Soil, a comparatively shallow deposit upon the surface of the earth, can in some places be easily washed away by heavy rains. Land thus robbed of its soil is sterile. In many countries, improvident handling, or should we say *lack* of handling the soil, has wrought havoc. Billions of tons of fertile soil have been washed into the rivers and seas and oceans. Countries which once supported teeming populations and boasted great wealth are now impoverished. Only a semblance of past productivity remains. Yet in an ancient Himalayan civilization a primitive people have, by constructing terraces, protected their soil and made it flourish.

The earth has about two and a half billion people who must be fed. The majority of this food must come from the soil, but the amount of soil is limited. Some may argue that we can always turn to the sea for sustenance, but could man actually live on sea products alone? I doubt it.

You cannot shrug and say "soil is soil" any more than you can say "man is man." There is a *mélange* of factors which enter into the picture. Just as a pregnant woman can only produce as healthy an infant as she is healthy, the soil can only be as fertile as its location and tenders permit it to be. For this reason, the desirability of location figures greatly in the grade value of land.

Mastery of the soil and of its enemies and the enemies of crop production is one of the greatest tasks facing future generations.

Dr. William A. Albrecht of the University of Missouri has said:

> We have often been told that "armies march on their stomachs." We have not been told that stomachs march according to the fertility of the soil. The fertility of the soil consists of those chemical elements of rock origin that contribute to the construction and body functions of both plants and animals.
>
> The human species may be reduced to a very simple basis. Man is about 5 percent soil, or 5 percent ash. This represents the soil's contribution to the construction of the body. The list of elements coming from the soil includes calcium, which makes up 1.6 percent of the normal body weight. Thus in a body of 150 pounds there is the equivalent in slaked lime required to lay a half-dozen bricks. The next element is phosphorus. This makes up 0.9 percent, or about one-third pounds per adult. The other elements of soil origin come in the following order: potassium 0.4, sodium 0.3, sulphur 0.2, magnesium 0.05, and iron 0.004 percent. There are traces of iodine, fluorine, silica, manganese, and others.

CHEMICAL ANALYSIS OF THE HUMAN BODY IN COMPARISON
WITH THAT OF PLANTS AND SOILS

	Human Body	Vegetation Dry Matter	Soil Dry Matter
Oxygen	66.0	42.9	47.3
Carbon	17.5	44.3	0.19
Hydrogen	10.2A	6.1A	0.22A
Nitrogen	2.4A	1.62A	—
Calcium	1.6A	0.62A	3.47A
Phosphorus	0.9A	0.56A	0.12A
Potassium	0.4A	1.68A	2.46A
Sodium	0.3	0.43	—
Chlorine	0.3	0.22	0.06
Sulphur	0.2	0.37	0.12
Magnesium	0.5	0.38	2.24
Iron	0.004	0.04	4.50
Iodine	—	Trace	—
Fluorine	—	Trace	0.10
Silicon	Trace	0 to 3.00	27.74
Manganese	—	Trace	0.08
Water	65.0	—	—
Protein	15.0	10.0	—
Carbohydrates	—	82.0	—
Fat	14.0	3.00	—
Salts	5.0	5.0	—
Other	1.0	—	—

From Dr. Albrecht's table it is evident that plants require the same elements as animals. It is also of great importance to note: "An adult body contains many soil elements. Life without any of them becomes impossible."

In 1946, Great Britain seemed to be undergoing a nutritional upheaval. Such published works remain today to substantiate this:

> Have starch-stuffed Britons come out of the war as physically fit as nutrition experts say? Many Britons doubt it. In the *London Observer*, commonsensical Air Chief Marshal Sir Philip Joubert quarreled with nutrition statistics that "confuse existence with life." He argued: "One can exist on the fruitless, starchy, dismal diet of Britain today, but what matters is liveliness, vitality, vigor. We are being led on to make a tremendous industrial effort. . . . That needs live folk, not mere existers."

More specific was the charge of Dr. Elizabeth Courley, a London school doctor. She said: "We have never had so many multiple boils, sores, rashes and scurvy. . . . With regard to Vitamin C, we have been reduced to an almost eighteenth-century plight."

In December 1945 in the United States Soil Conservation Service publications the following statements were made:

> The U.S. produces more food than any other nation in the world, yet, according to Dr. Thomas Parran, Jr., 40 percent of the population suffers from malnutrition. How can this be true? The majority of the people get enough to eat. Evidently the food eaten does not have enough of the right minerals and vitamins in it to keep them healthy. What causes food to lack these necessary elements? Investigators have found that food is no richer in minerals than the soil from which it comes. Depleted soils will not produce healthy nutritious plants. Plants suffering from mineral deficiencies will not nourish healthy animals. Mineral-deficient plants and undernourished animals will not support our people in health. Poor soils perpetuate poor people physically, mentally, and financially.

The human body requires twelve major elements and a number of trace elements to function properly. Take away any one of these elements and normal life cannot exist. Investigators have demonstrated that the quantitative variations of such inorganic elements as calcium, phosphorus, iodine, copper, cobalt and iron in foods and feeds are very important factors in human and animal health. It is known that when soils of an area lack iodine, the people living in that area do not receive enough in the locally grown food and therefore suffer a high incidence of goiter. It was found in certain districts in Florida, where the predominant soils were classified as deficient in iron, copper and cobalt, that from 52 to 96 percent of the children were anemic. Dietary deficiencies are rarely single and specific in effect, as in the case of goiter and anemia, but cover a wide range of disturbed body functions that we ordinarily overlook and do not think of as being caused by the mineral deficiencies of our soils.

In some localities, animals born in the early winter develop rickets by late winter or early spring due to calcium and phosphorus deficiencies. Cows suffering from this deficiency cannot get sufficient minerals from their grazing grasses to develop their bones.

In the development of their offspring, they have to draw so heavily on the minerals of their own bodies that the bones in their horns and tails are completely used up.

Crop-juggling is no permanent substitute for soil deficiencies. New plants that will produce better growth on mineral-deficient soil can be brought in, but analyses of these plants show that they, too, are deficient in the same minerals as the soil on which they are grown.

Land should contain the right minerals for developing brains, brawn and character. All we are, and all we wish to be—with the exception of our spiritual and genetic heritage—comes from what we eat, drink and breathe. The theory concerning soil and its importance to good nutrition is no longer theory but fact. The soil in which our food is raised is of the greatest importance to us if we wish to maintain good health, intelligence and character.

Why do the best trotting horses come from Kentucky? Simply because Kentucky is world-famous for its "sky-high" Bluegrass—Bluegrass grown in certain sections which have magnificent soil conditions containing the needed minerals, such as potassium, phosphorus, iron, iodine, calcium and magnesium.

There are a number of farms all over the country now, and especially in Southern California, where the soil has been enriched with minerals and humus. The protein content of alfalfa grown on such land has increased, and the animals grazed on such fields have given superior dairy products. Plants grown on such soil stay healthy, free from insects and do not require poison sprays. The same applies to fruits, grains and vegetables.

Although as yet only a tiny number have been converted to follow this health pattern of soil conservation, many U. S. scientists and teachers have been dreaming of a luscious and rich soil for America, of creating a Shangri-la—following in the footsteps of the Hunza people. They and a number of others are trying to help the farmers grow better food and protect their soils.

In fact a group of physicians, dentists, and laymen met in Chicago in 1950 and formed the "Natural Food Associates," as a non-profit organization under the leadership of Joe D. Nichols, a surgeon in Atlanta, Texas. Their objectives are to educate all people to the value of poison-free natural food grown on fertile soil. . . . And to tell them how and where to get this food. Also they help any farmer who asks for help to improve the conditions of his soil.

They publish a monthly magazine *National Food and Farming* which contains articles on organic gardening.

In giving Americans nutritious foods we will lay the foundation for health, strength, stamina, integrity and love. The oneness of the body, mind and spirit is an integral part of life and cannot be separated. The Hunzakuts, because of their healthy bodies, have achieved spiritual heights and have become the most peaceful people on earth. They have done it and we can do it, too. Each individual has to build the urge and understanding within himself to improve these conditions. One individual represents a family, a state, a nation. Then peace might descend upon us as it has in Hunza for over 130 years. The soil is the source of all life, the starting point in human health.

15.

Hunza
Magic

Hunza is a friendly place. The Hunzakuts have understanding hearts and warm dispositions. They are a happy people.

In spite of their primitive surroundings and lack of so-called modern education, they are unusually well balanced emotionally and have learned to live peacefully within their communities and with others outside their realm.

The people of Hunza have a genuine respect for the rights of others. This was demonstrated during court sessions when water rights were involved. How simply such problems were solved by mutual understanding and heart-to-heart talks!

Much of our difficulty in relationships arises from the fact that we tend to form hasty opinions of others and jump to conclusions. Some of us find fault with others and fail to discover our true relationship to each other. Many persons have unintentionally cultivated a critical outlook on life in general. This is a wrong mental attitude which only reflects our own conditions and brings bitterness and unhappiness into our lives.

The Hunzakuts, on the other hand, are positive thinkers. Every job is done without worrying ahead of time whether it can be done. The people of Hunza have faith in God and believe He is an unseen partner in all of their undertakings.

We, too, apply this same attitude in various instances, but not often enough. For instance, a pilot who takes a plane from New York to Los Angeles says, "In four and a half hours we shall be in Los Angeles." He does not say, "If everything goes well, we shall reach Los Angeles." The pilot assumes a positive attitude and doesn't allow any doubts to creep into his mind.

If we foresee trouble, that is what we get. If we envision success, harmony, health and abundance, we experience these conditions in our lives. Since our thoughts are the invisible builders of our destiny, we should be careful about the kind of thoughts we allow to enter our consciousness. If we find negative thoughts intruding, we must throw them out at once and replace them with constructive thoughts. We are either strengthening or weakening our universe each day by the kind of thoughts we entertain. We are also building or destroying our health and vigor in the same way.

Dr. Frank N. Allan, a Boston internist, in his study of three hundred victims of chronic exhaustion, found that only 20 percent were tired for purely physical reasons, while 80 percent were tired because of emotional difficulties.

> A study of chronically tired business executives in their early forties and fifties was made at a Chicago hospital. These men had been full of driving ambition, eager to accept responsibilties, determined to reach the top. But somewhere along the way they had lost their drive, their incentive to work. All were thoroughly discouraged and terribly tired. "It seemed that their mainsprings were broken," observed one physician.*

That is very well put—"their mainsprings were broken." The Hunzakuts are constantly building up their internal strength and stamina instead of destroying it with negative emotions.

Extreme exhaustion is our common complaint. We push and push, afraid to stop, and this fear drives us to desperation. All is caused by lack of a positive attitude, positive thinking. When we do something because we believe in it, because we want to do it, and we feel in advance that it will be a success, no fear creeps into our subconscious to destroy our energy and make us tired.

The people of Hunza go on working without apparent fatigue. It

*In an article, "*How to Live Without Fatigue*," in *The Reader's Digest*, condensed from *Why So Tired*, by Marguerite Clark.

is amazing to watch them working or playing, or even just walking. They don't walk, they glide. The Mir told me his messenger prefers to walk to Gilgit, 68 miles distant, rather than ride a horse. However, I still believe that some sort of transportation is preferable for that distance, although the Hunzakuts don't agree with me.

People who are positive thinkers cannot succumb to worry, for they know that Worry is a ravenous creature who, in this great and teeming world, has chewed a solid niche for himself into our society. If allowed to run his helter-skelter course through the human body, he will succeed in destroying its source—or mainspring—of strength. He has a way of corkscrewing himself into the lining of intestines until, in some cases, lesions known as an ulcer develop. With his willful ways, Worry can induce heartburn, nausea, loss of appetite, diarrhea, pimples, hives, rashes of various dimensions and colors and, as is often the case in the constant rush of the business world, he can also induce a nervous breakdown. He can whittle his way into the subconscious mind so that the individual becomes totally unable to deal with circumstances which arise around him. Worry fixes it so that the slightest thing, such as the change of weather or a grating sound, can become such an irritant that the body in whom he dwells is reduced to tears and tyrannical shoutings.

The above portrait of Worry is not exaggerated. Worry exists and it is up to each of us to begin to wage a private war against him.

God created man in His own image and invested him with many qualities and abilities, among them the spiritual power to fulfill his purpose on earth. He has given us all we need to achieve a happy life, establish peace, health, harmony, abundance and order. Worry, however, is an intruder obviously sent from the wrong side of the tracks. Worry is indeed a wetback who stealthily waded his way across the River Styx one dark night to invade the realm of mankind. He has succeeded in infiltrating every nation save one, the land of Hunza. In Hunza, men and women live without Worry.

Mental exercises are just as essential as physical exercises and, if we intend to execute Worry, we must practice day by day. We must develop faith and strength by putting them to work, just as we develop muscles by continuous use.

We may not see immediate or outward results, but they will come. Turn your efforts into constructive channels, and if the imps of negation nudge your consciousness you must bar them by placing positive thoughts in their path. A negative and a positive thought mix about as well as oil and water.

When we worry, we are possessed by negativeness, and we borrow trouble unnecessarily, for we look ahead into the future and try to see the storms of life approaching. Naturally we distress ourselves long before anything serious happens, and so when a crisis, even a small one, arises we are already in such a state of anxiety that we can hardly cope with it. Not until you learn to relax can you rid yourself of Worry. Tensions of the mind are passed on to the body, and these tensions can cause physical as well as mental disorders.

Dr. Hans Selye has said:

> We are just beginning to see that many common diseases are due largely to errors in our adaptive responses to stress, rather than to direct damage by germs, poisons, or other external agents. In this sense, many nervous and emotional disturbances, high blood pressure, gastric and duodenal ulcers, certain types of rheumatic, cardiovascular and renal diseases, appear to be essentially diseases of adaptation. In view of all this, stress is undoubtedly an important personal problem for everyone.*

Childhood diseases (mumps, measles, chicken pox, etc.) do not exist in Hunza. In the entire modern history of peace-ruled Hunza, not one individual has suffered from an ulcer. The Hunzakuts are living proof of Dr. Selye's theories. Fear, stress and almost all forms of anxiety are foreign to these wonderful people.

Dr. Selye says:

> The secret of health lies in the successful adjustment to changing stresses. The penalty for failure in this great process of adaptation is ill-health and unhappiness. Stress is essentially the mate of all the wear-and-tear caused by life. Although we cannot avoid stress as long as we live, we can learn how to keep its damaging side-effects to a minimum. Stress is not any deviation from the steady state of the body.

The Hunza people have developed a highly positive attitude toward life. One day while the Mir and I were discussing their problem of lack of land, he calmly said, "Well, if a mountain is in

* Quote from an article, *"Remaking Your Idea,"* by Hans Selye, M.D. *Vogue,* January 15, 1957.

our way, we will simply have to move it!" And he was not jesting, he spoke completely in earnest. I have no doubt that should the need arise to "move that mountain," the Mir and his people will find a way to do it.

Watching the faces of the Hunzakuts, you see happy smiles and expressions of confidence and self-assurance. A wonderful feeling of peace prevails in Hunza: a feeling attained only when Worry has been exorcised, a feeling of a direct contact with God. Peace, harmony and well-being of spirit are enjoyed here, for the Hunzakuts are free from the regrets of the past and apprehensions about the future. They carry out their daily chores quietly, without stress or strain, without nervous tension. Therefore, when the job is completed, it is done well and efficiently.

We redecorate our homes, buy new clothes, new furniture or a new car, but I wonder how many of us ever consider redecorating our mental house? Whether we like to accept it or not, we look at the world through the windows of our own mentalities. We interpret everything we see in terms of our own mental limitations. Fortunately, however, we can transform our lives and our circumstances through the spiritual process of renewing our thoughts, and by continually redecorating the house of our minds.

Our thoughts are the tools we use in carving our lives. Man is made or unmade by himself, and life can only give back what we put into it. Noble character is not a thing of chance, it is the result of continued effort in right thinking, and by the same process, ignoble character is the result of continually harboring base thoughts. Truly, man molds his own character, and if he wishes a change, he and he alone can bring about that change.

Let us sever mental connections with the trouble-monger Worry and learn to live life gloriously, concentrating all our ambitions on the "things of good repute" which we wish to experience and accomplish.

Let us look to the Hunzakuts. There is no greed, no jealousy, no envy and no false attitudes to poison their minds and hearts. They have faith in God and a true love for one another. They do not put the blame for their problems on fate or bad luck or on anyone or anything other than themselves and their own thinking processes. It is obvious that we, too, must adopt their marvelous and simple plan for cooperative existence.

The people of Hunza can show us the way to happiness if we

will only let them. Nowhere in the world are there happier people. There is a purpose in their every movement and in their every job. You may argue that they work only to exist, that they do not desire money or things of great material value, simply because they have never known luxury. Perhaps! But does luxury and wealth constitute happiness and prosperity? I think not. How many millionaires do you find on pleasure cruises confessing that they are sailing the seven seas in search of happiness and in search of themselves? In Hunza, life's work brings a much greater paycheck than money. It brings contentment. The Hunzakuts have found happiness and prosperity—prosperity in the true riches of life: love, peace of mind, health and spiritual understanding. There are no neurotics in Hunza. They have built a pattern of thought which has created a satisfying, purposeful life.

Our problems, our amusements and our work occupy our minds so completely that relaxation to so many of us is impossible without tranquilizers. There is no longer any room in our existence for quietude. We say we clamor for it, but when we achieve it we don't know what to do with it. In Hunza, people find time to meditate in the silence of their homes or in the little mosques which stand in each village. Twice daily, first thing in the morning and just before retiring, each Hunzakut takes the time to say a quiet prayer and to meditate for a few moments. Actually the Hunzakuts are a unique example of Christianity in action. They practice everything Christ taught. "Love thy neighbor as thyself," is their creed. It is amazing to watch the people of Hunza as they exercise faith in everything they do. Every move is based on their faith in God. When we were in the mountains on the road to Hunza, no matter what hardship developed the Hunzakuts were confident that no harm could possibly come to them. They smiled and laughed and sang and kept up an optimistic mood. Their spirit and positive attitude helped the members of our expedition to gain courage to withstand all the difficulties which lay before us.

Faith is the rock upon which the great institutions of mankind have been built. Faith is stronger than presumption. It is stronger than credulity. It carries one far beyond prospect and chance. Faith transcends hope and fulfills expectation.

Remember, that in order to live we must live for today, for now. This is the only time in which we live when we can truthfully say "I *am*." What is life if our time is always a moment which is expected to arise somewhere in the not-too-distant future! What is life if we fail to live *this* moment joyfully and radiantly! Gather together the ragged edges of worry and skepticism and weave them into a pattern of joy and serenity.

The people of Hunza have shown us a fabric of great worth: the fabric of self-assurance and positive thinking. In Hunza there is no room for pettiness or jealousy. There is no such thing as that "why do you have more than I do" feeling. Gratitude exists in every heart—the gratitude to God for creating them. Love echoes in everyone's mind. Love cannot destroy. It can only create, and where there is love there can be no fear.

16.

The Secret Path
to Happiness

Before I actually traveled to Hunza, I had been studying the land and its people for close to a decade. In whatever I read about this tiny kingdom of everlasting health, the importance of their food and exercise was stressed to the point of excluding any mention of their spiritual and emotional qualities.

While there, I was able to learn something about the spiritual side of Hunza life. In fact, "learn" is really the wrong word—I merely needed to observe. The Hunzakuts live what they believe more than any other group of people in the world. Their level of spiritual development never ceases to amaze me. Mentally and spiritually, their practice of the principles of their religion is without exception. Religion is not something that is read about, something that sermons are preached about. No, to them religion is a way of life, and they live their religion during every wakeful moment of their lives. When you hear that there are no jails, no crimes of passion, no juvenile delinquency and no police in this nation, you are certainly astounded, but after witnessing their way of life you realize that there is nothing startling about this lack of crime. It is the natural result of their approach to life, the actual living principles of all the texts of religion, the Bible, the Koran and the Talmud. In Hunza you can observe the actions of self-sacrifice, of tenderness and of brotherly love, all the inspiring messages of the great religious texts are demonstrated here by these simple God-loving people.

There is a great lesson to be learned from the history of this group of people. In the early periods of their growth they were brigands, a warlike nation, committed to raids upon the rich caravans that passed their way. It was a wild, self-satisfying life in every sense of the word. But somewhere in the distant past they decided that fighting and killing were negative aspects of life, that there were many wonderful values in life that they were missing. Within a few years they became a peaceful nation of brotherly love.

The lesson they demonstrated is simple: *it can be done*. People can shake off a heritage of greed, jealousy and power. The people of Hunza have demonstrated that love, brotherhood and a spiritually inspired life bring happiness. They are a living example of what so many of our humanistic leaders have been telling us: when we truly learn to understand each other, to fulfill the precepts of brotherly love, to live simply, then we will find that utopia of a community in which all the promises of the religions of the world will find their rewarding fulfillment.

I am convinced that only purity of soil, purity of mind and the desire to live in brotherhood can save the future. This is the lesson of the people of Hunza—the living Shangri-la. They long ago learned that only in love, harmony, health and happiness can humanity survive and prosper.

As for us, there is still time—time to face this truth: "In vain do we build the City if we do not first build the Man."

For the first time in my life I felt that I truly had a purpose in living. And if the message of love, faith, peace and long life can benefit our way of life . . . then all the anxiety and dangers connected with my journey have been worthwhile.

Faith is a wonderful thing. It is the very substance of things hoped for. It stirs the mind to hold to the belief that all things are possible. As the Master promised, "According to your faith be it done unto you." Faith is a vital power, and it is up to us to direct our faith in a constructive channel.

Faith and courage ar two great possessions, never let them go away from you. Someone said: "Courage is man's greatest strength and the ready companion of unshakable faith!"

17.
Vitamins
You Should
Know About

In a previous chapter, I discussed the values of minerals and foods containing the specific ones. Now I would like to write about individual vitamins with reference to the function each must perform if the body is to grow normally, and keep well.

The diet on which the Hunza people have lived for a long time is no doubt responsible for the good health they enjoy. A balanced natural diet should supply us with all the proteins, vitamins, minerals and enzymes our bodies need. And yet, serious deficiencies exist among our population.

This is so because some of our foods are picked before they are ripe, and thus are robbed of the vitamin values resulting from appropriate and necessary sun-ripening. Then they are stored in dark, cold refrigerator cars to be transported to the cities and finally to market. A substantial percentage of vitamins and trace elements is lost through the lack of sun and abnormal temperature. Even before harvesting and shipping, much food suffers further deprivation of nutrients from depleted soil and the use of harmful sprays. In the final processing of some foods, all nutritive value is destroyed by the addition of preservatives and other unnatural ingredients. In sum, vitamins, minerals and enzymes, in tablet form, are often essential to supplement our diet.

173

And since vitamins are derived from food, it makes sense to seek out natural sources as much as possible.

Vitamin A. Vitamin A is needed for normal eyesight in dim light. It is necessary also for growth and for healthy teeth, bones, nerves and good skin. It can be found in bright yellow fruits and vegetables such as cantaloupes, carrots, apricots, squash, tomatoes and all leafy green vegetables; liver, butter, eggs, as well as fish oil, whole milk, cream and cheeses. It can be stored in the body. It is not water soluble; therefore it should be taken in moderation or on your doctor's advice.

The Vitamin B Complex Family.

The B complex is primarily involved with nervous systems; a deficiency might cause nervous tension and irritability but could also result in baldness or anemia or acne or any of a number of physical and mental illnesses still being discovered as linked to the B complex.

a) B-1, or *thiamine*. The richest source is found in wheat germ and rice polish, but thiamine can also be found in brewer's yeast, cereal grains, nuts, legumes and unrefined foods prepared from seeds such as peanut butter, breads and cereals. Among animal sources of B-1 are kidney and heart.

b) B-2, or *riboflavin*. B-2 contributes to a healthy skin, bright eyes and calm nerves. Foods richest in vitamin B-2 are milk, cottage cheese, yogurt, eggs, meat and liver as well as green leafy vegetables, almonds, soybeans, brewer's yeast, avocados and peas.

c) B-3, or *niacin*. An insufficient amount of this vitamin might cause problems ranging from insomnia to pellagra and include poor digestion and fatigue. Its richest sources are skim-milk powder, brewer's yeast, fish, liver, wheat germ, molasses and soya flour.

d) B-6, or *pyridoxine*. B-6 must be supplied daily. It is particularly important in mental health, skin disorders, overweight (it acts as a natural diuretic), and nerve disorders such as Parkinson's disease. It also helps in the metabolism of fats. B-6 can be found in liver, brewer's yeast, wheat germ, whole grains, soybeans, nuts, egg yolks, skim-milk powder and green vegetables.

e) B-12. B-12 is one of the most essential of all the vitamins, and has been found to be effective against anemia and many diseases of the nerves. It is needed in very small amounts and when found to be a serious need, is often given by injection. It is found in muscle meats, kidney, egg yolks, milk, yogurt, wheat germ and—primarily—liver. It is the B vitamin not contained in brewer's yeast; however, many suppliers are now adding B-12 to brewer's yeast so that the whole complex is available in it.

Inositol. Inositol is an important nutrient for cell membranes and bone marrow; it is needed for healthy growth of the hair. It is assumed that we can get enough of this vitamin from our food, but this assumption is not correct unless the daily diet is rich in liver, brewer's yeast, fruits, nuts, skim-milk powder, soybeans, and whole grains.

Choline. This is one of the "lipotropic" or fat-splitting factors and is an important vitamin for the liver. It helps to remove fats from the liver and to distribute them throughout the body to places where they can be utilized. Best foods are wheat germ and legumes.

Pantothenic acid. This powerful B vitamin is effective against stress and is needed for the formation of certain hormones. It helps the body achieve general good health. It is found in liver and other organ meats, egg yolk, broccoli, cauliflower, brewer's yeast.

Para-aminobenzoic acid. PABA is essential for the normal functioning of the glands. Foods such as brewer's yeast, rice polish and liver are rich in this vitamin.

Folic acid. An aid in the manufacture of red blood cells, folic acid is essential in normal metabolism—the converting of food to energy. It is found in liver, navy beans, dark green leafy vegetables, nuts, fresh oranges, whole wheat products.

Biotin. Biotin assists in the burning up of fatty acids and carbohydrates for body heat and energy. It is found in organ meats, whole grain and brewer's yeast.

Vitamin C. This vitamin is also known as ascorbic acid. An adequate amount must be taken daily because this essential nutrient is not stored in the body. It is vital for the firmness and health of gums and teeth; it helps to guard against infections of all kinds and insures the health of the connective tissues which cushion the bones and joints. Vitamin C is also necessary in the healing of broken bones. All fresh, growing foods contain vitamin C; nevertheless, citrus fruits, guavas, ripe bell peppers and pimentos, and the seed pods of wild roses, known as rose hips, are its richest sources.

Vitamin D. This is a two-way vitamin which may be obtained from foods and from sunshine. It is necessary for good bones and teeth. It promotes the body's use of calcium. Vitamin D, when taken in excess of the daily requiremen's, may be stored in the liver for future use. It is also stored in the livers of many fish; in fact, fish-liver products such as cod-liver oil, halibut-liver oil and perch are our richest sources. Babies and young children need a special supply of this vitamin regularly. Other sources of vitamin D are irradiated yeast, tuna, herring and mackerel.

Vitamin E. Vitamin E is valuable to the function of every cell in the body but especially to the heart and circulating system. It is also a highly efficient treatment for burns and scar tissue and is recognized as an important nutrient in pregnancy. It has long been known as the anti-sterility vitamin and is used to relieve menopause symptoms. Most of the vitamin E is discarded from grains when flours are refined. It can be found in wheat germ, wheat germ oil and whole grains, green vegetables and dairy products.

Vitamin K. This vitamin need not be of concern to a healthy person whose diet is adequate in milk and unsaturated fatty acids and low in refined carbohydrates. Foods rich in vitamin K are cabbage, cauliflower, spinach and all leafy vegetables, beet tops, tops of carrots, kale, Swiss chard and alfalfa.

18.

Any Questions?
I'll Be Happy
to Answer Them

It is always a delight for me to answer questions about the Hunza people during the question and answer periods which always end my lectures and personal appearances. And the questions are many, believe me, for this wonderful land and its beautiful people are endlessly fascinating to everyone. Here are some typical questions I am asked:

Q. Have you a film on Hunza?

A. Yes, I have several films which were all made on location. In fact, an educational-documentary film produced in 1977 is available for rent or sale. It is a 30-minute, 16mm, color film which won the Award of Excellence from the Film Advisory Board.

Q. Can we write to you for more information about Hunza?

A. Yes—and every letter will be answered—but help me get to your letter promptly by sending a self-addressed, stamped reply envelope.

Q. What do the Hunza people eat as a rule?

A. In the previous chapters I discussed foods and things they grow. However, this question is asked frequently, so I shall answer it again. They eat millet, wheat, buckwheat and barley; vegetables such as turnips, carrots, potatoes, corn, peas, beans and leafy vegetables; also cucumbers and a variety of squashes; some meat (usually mutton and chicken); milk products and fruits such as apricots, peaches, apples, pears, grapes, mulberries and a variety of melons—most of them have different flavors from ours. At times, a glass of local grape wine accompanies a meal.

Q. How does death come?

A. One day the oldster is there; the next he is gone. The Mir expressed it in these words: "We *expire*. One is tired and wants to get some rest."

Q. How large are their families?

A. As arable land and consequent food production is limited in Hunza, families are kept small, to two or three children.

Q. Do Hunza women outlive their men as is customary in other countries?

A. The contrary is true in Hunza. Men outlive the women by an average of about ten to twenty years.

Q. Do they have divorces?

A. The Hunzakuts have tranquil dispositions and from early childhood they are taught how to get along with others. Divorce is rare.

Q. How do Hunza women dress?

A. Costumes of native women are somewhat like those worn by gypsies. They are gaudy with color.

Q. Does their water have any minerals in it?

A. Hunza water comes from mountain streams fed by melting ice and snow high in the mountains. Passing over and through rocks and soil, the water picks up valuable minerals which are deposited as silt on the fields during irrigation periods. The water is dark gray in color, and the natives prefer this dark water for drinking purposes. Foreigners generally drink water that has been allowed to settle, and looks clear. I adopted the native custom and found the water delicious.

Q. Do they employ commercial fertilizers and insecticides?

A. Commercial fertilizers are forbidden by law. The fertility of the soil is superior because only natural elements are used to enrich it. Everything that is taken from the soil is returned to the soil. As pests are negligible, insecticides are unnecessary.

Q. Can we import food from Hunza?

A. No. Hunza does not have sufficient food to permit export; besides, our laws prevent it. There is no canning of fruits and vegetables in Hunza.

Q. Do they have money?

A. Hunza does not have a national currency. They use Pakistani money, since they are a state of Pakistan. However, the people have very little money, and they transact such business as they do mostly by barter.

Q. What would you say is the best philosophy of life to follow?
A. Think young . . . feel young . . . act young—the way the Hunzas do, and you will find the road to Eternal Youth. According to an old Moslem proverb:

> The Man who has Health has Hope,
> And who has Hope, has Everything.

19.

From
the Hunzas
for Today

The story you have just read is not a work of fiction. It is real—magnificent, inspiring Hunza, the land of eternal peace and beauty; the land of such harmony and serenity that all the modern world should pause and gaze at it with awe, bewilderment, and complete respect.

In an age when the threat of global thermonuclear war hovers over this planet like an impending shroud, perhaps it would be wise to look back at the road which the Hunzakuts have traveled in the past. As we have learned, in the old days the economy there depended upon raids made by local bandits upon the unsuspecting caravans crossing the Himalayas from Kashmir and China en route to India. Captured enemies were sold into slavery and murder was commonplace as the members of the royal families battled for power.

This was the Hunza of old. But somehow out of this destructiveness and brutality, the people of Hunza blindly stumbled onto that all-too-elusive road to peace.

As I go back to visit Hunza each time, I witness some changes, made in gradual, simple steps that do not disorient the people, nor attack their social structures, their self-confidence, their age-old spiritual values and wisdom. But change is *life*, and recognizing this, Hunza is getting ready for today's world. They have a great message—a priceless gift for modern humanity which is ready to receive it more than ever before. It is the message of peace and hope, an experience every man and woman would want to share.

This is not the first change for the Hunza people. From an origin of unprincipled existence evolved the spiritually serene life of Hunza society today. The roots of this culture might remind us of a portion of the dilemma of our modern-world-inner-city crime, weakened political leadership, greed, lust and fear. Let us learn from them about changing into the garment of peace and happiness.

The Hunzakuts have found happiness and prosperity —prosperity in the true riches of life: love, peace of mind, health and spiritual understanding. There are no neurotics in Hunza. Besides, they are well organized: they work hard, nevertheless, they find time for recreation, rest, and meditation twice a day in the silence of their homes or out in the open air. It is amazing to watch the people of Hunza as they exercise faith in everything they do.

Somehow, most of us live in a state of spiritual amnesia. We allow our physical senses to rule our existence, and destroy the pleasures and joys of real life. Even sex has been abused and turned into an ugly performance. Sex is a great art, and should be treated with care, love and mutual understanding; only then, can two people experience to the fullest satisfaction the bodily need for sex.

We cannot expect to have mental coordination and a body brimming with health and spiritual beauty by leading a careless and chaotic life. Our thoughts and actions must become harmonious. Drugs, smoking, alcohol in excess are used because people are unhappy. Our society is becoming more and more complex.

I must admit that the importance of physical exercise and proper nutrition is gaining momentum today. There still is much to be done to make everyone aware of how much more pleasure one can derive by leading a life without pain and illness. How many can truly claim it!

The rest of the world, I feel, could profit from the wisdom of the Hunzakuts' way of life and practice of Yoga. A well-planned program combining the simple Hunza diet with a few yoga exercises, would be a perfect formula for daily living.

My theories have been born of long practice and study of the Hunza way of life and yoga techniques and philosophy. I have lived among the amazing people of Hunza. I watched them work and play; I have eaten their food. I have also studied and taught yoga for many years. The combination of the two seems to be logical. Practising the yoga method of deep rhythmic breathing, exercise and relaxation, man can strengthen his body, which in turn will strengthen his mind and spirit. And simple, nutritive foods build healthier organs, blood and cells.

I observed students who followed such a program and noticed that it not only changed their outward appearance, it made them grow spiritually into wonderful human beings.

Tension is the cause of our society's many problems, including the teenage use of drugs. I am eager to reach as many people as possible, young and old alike. I am convinced yoga and proper nutrition can begin the discipline of emotions.

I taught yoga to a group of students at one of the colleges in my area and the results were tremendous. Most of them gave up smoking and taking drugs. It strengthens my belief that young people as well as adults who take drugs can be helped through a definite program.

So many times during my public appearances or in my classes, inevitably, the question comes up: "Why did you become interested in Hunza?" It all began in New York. I went to hear a German doctor, M.O. Garten, whose subject was Hunza—the healthiest people on earth. From him I learned that Hunza was not a myth; it existed and its people claimed perfect health and longevity. Out of curiosity I asked the doctor: "Do you think any one in our society doing the same things they do, can get well or keep well?" "Of course," he answered with a grin, "but people in our society have no faith and don't even try. It is much easier to complain and feel sorry for oneself."

My personal health at that time was at stake. I was failing rapidly. Treatments and medicine were of no help, and it had been pronounced that an operation was unavoidable. I made up my mind, without any hesitation, to try the Hunza way of Life. If the theory works and I get well, I promised myself, I would devote the rest of my life to helping others. I followed it step-by-step: first I went on a fast, and gave up smoking, then stopped eating junk foods and began to exercise, walking and even reorganizing my thinking. Soon I looked forward to every living day. Indeed, it was a new and delightful experience. It happened in 1953 and I have had enjoyed Life ever since.

My books were born based on personal experience. Since my first trip to Hunza in 1961 I have written several on nutrition and yoga. *Hunza Health Secrets*, first published in 1964, has brought joy and new experiences to hundreds of thousands of people all over this country and around the world, since it has been published in several countries in foreign languages.

Then I wrote *Yoga . . . the Art of Living*, (the original title in hard cover was *The Hunza-Yoga Way to Health and Longer Life*). *Hunza . . . the Himalayan Shangri-la*, and *Come Along to Hunza*, are the history of these people, illustrated with many pictures, original copies of the royal family's private collection. The Mir and I worked on the history together to make sure all the facts were correct and authentic.

The Palace was also my home while I was there and it gave me the opportunity to learn to know the royal family well, and to love them dearly.

So often the question was asked: "What is the life of a Queen like? And what happens during the day inside the palace?"

To satisfy your curiosity I will draw you a picture of a typical day of the Rani (the Queen) and the other members of the royal family. Her day starts officially at six o'clock when she joins her husband the Mir in the dining room for breakfast. However, they both get up much earlier to devote time to quiet devotion separately. The Mir prays from the Koran, their Bible, at the tomb of his beloved grandfather, Nazim Khan, whilst the Rani meditates in the seclusion of her private chambers.

Breakfast doesn't consist of much food. Herb tea and fresh fruit are typical. For the visitors a choice of eggs and the local bread (chapatti) freshly baked are served on demand. The native people don't eat much in the morning.

When the Mir leaves for his office, the Rani begins her job. She plans with the chef the meals for the day, then she assigns duties to the numerous household crew. There is no commotion; every one listens quietly and then leaves the room to attend to their chores.

Lunch is served at one o'clock. A soup prepared of herbs was a favorite of mine. The mint herbs especially tasted so delicate. Then rice-spinach or lamb curry as a main dish. Meat is not too often served as the small pastures cannot feed too many heads of cattle. A salad, consisting of freshly picked lettuce, cucumbers, radishes and some herbs, is always served with salad dressing, a combination of apricot kernel oil and grape vinegar, prepared at the table by everyone to taste. Then there are always freshly baked chapattis.

The Rani is an excellent hostess and an expert in superb cuisine. She takes pride in serving delicious food in her home. I learned to prepare most of the Hunza dishes under her supervision.

After lunch the Rani retires to her room to rest. At five o'clock she entertains on the glassed-in veranda. All the women of the palace household with their children, the daughters and the English governess, gather together. Tea and a variety of home-made pastries with fresh fruit fillings, dried apricots, and nuts are served.

It was obvious to me that the servants felt at ease in the presence of their Queen and spoke without hesitation in their Hunza language. The royal family speaks perfect English. Then the chef, who has been taught to cook by the Rani herself, joins the group for a short while to report about his department. The children behave so very well, no one is aware of their presence.

By seven o'clock everyone quietly leaves to get ready for dinner at nine'clock. For the evening meal everyone dresses in formal attire. Again the whole family (but this time all the men are present) gathers on the veranda. Sparkling Hunza-made wine from grapes is served.

At exactly nine o'clock the gong rings for dinner and everyone follows the Queen into the dining room. She always leads the way inside of her house. The long table is set with silver and fine rare china. Spaced along its length are silver candelabra supporting a glistening array of pure white candles. The royal insignia is embroidered in gold on each piece of linen. The sparkling silver, the shimmering light of the candles, the deep, rich colors of the plump fruit and the mirror-like surface of the hand-painted china give a festive, elegant air to the room.

The food is always excellent. A great variety of dishes include dessert and fresh fruit. One day, ice cream was served. Snow, pure white snow from the Himalayan glaciers sweetened with dried, pureed apricots, fooled all of us into believing it was ice-cream. A stack of steaming hot chapattis is a part of every meal.

After dinner everyone joins the Queen in the drawing room for a cup of tea. Then it is time to retire and the day comes to an end. A perfect day!

It has been said so many times: "A sound mind in a sound body." Obviously the ultimate aim of this book is to build a harmony and unity of body and mind and consciousness.

Life can have a perfect balance. In the last century man's average life span has increased to 75 years, but we could live much longer. To reach that state we have to give up some of our habits, such as smoking in excess; eating too much elaborate food; drinking alcohol and emotional stress and strain. Man has to acquire the knowledge of how to live a long life and to enjoy more fully the life he has now.

What is man? Is he the master of his fate? Can he conquer old age, disease and death? Man differs from other animals because he is endowed with a highly developed brain which directs the activities of his body. Man's brain allows him to think, to choose and to act. He is free to choose his own environment and actions, but he cannot foresee the results. Of course, if we don't search or study, we find nothing or experience nothing.

The disciplined self has a strong will and therefore the senses and mind obey the will. If the mind says: "I must get this or that," and if it is not the right thing for you to have, then say: "I won't cooperate with you today, you will not get this or that." The self-controlled man will not be distracted by objects, for his senses will choose the right road to achieve his goal.

It is essential to wipe out lust, greed and egoism, and entertain only positive thoughts, to close your mind to negative thoughts before they can damage your brain. The more you practice, the stronger you will grow spiritually. Fear, buried hatred, intolerance, anger, disturb the action of the subconscious mind. Instead, cultivate your virtues.

Whatever you sow by your actions comes back to you no matter what it is. Wilfred A. Peterson said: "Man alone of all the creatures of earth, can change his own pattern; man alone is architect of his destiny."

Renée Taylor
Redondo Beach, California
1978

Books to Read

These books can bring joy and enlightenment into your life.

Abrahamson, E. M., M.D., and Pezet, A. W. 1971. *Body, Mind and Sugar.* New York: Jove Books.

Carson, Rachel. 1962. *Silent Spring.* Greenwich, Connecticut: Fawcett Publications.

Clark, Linda. 1973. *Know Your Nutrition.* New Canaan, Connecticut: Keats Publishing, Inc.

Davis, Adelle. 1947. *Let's Cook It Right.* New York: New American Library.

Ellwood, Cathryn. *Feel Like a Million.* New York: Pocket Books

Fredericks, Carlton. 1975. *Look Younger, Feel Healthier.* New York: Grosset & Dunlap.

Hauser, Gayelord. 1976. *Gayelord Hauser's New Treasury of Secrets.* New York: Dell Publishers.

Hunter, Beatrice Trum. 1973. *Fact/Book on Additives and Your Health.* New Canaan, Connecticut: Keats Publishing, Inc.

Hunter, Beatrice Trum. 1966. *The Natural Foods Cookbook.* New York: Jove Books.

Lappé, Frances M. 1975. *Diet for a Small Planet.* New York: Ballantine Books.

Larson, Gena. 1972. *Better Foods for Better Babies and Their Families.* New Canaan, Connecticut: Keats Publishing, Inc.

Longgood, William. 1962. *The Poisons in Your Food.* New York: Jove Books.

Page, Melvin E. and Abrams, H. L. 1972. *Your Body Is Your Best Doctor.* New Canaan, Connecticut: Keats Publishing, Inc.

Pfeiffer, Carl C., M.D. 1975. *Mental and Elemental Nutrients.* New Canaan, Connecticut: Keats Publishing, Inc.

Rodale, J. I. 1954. *The Health Finder.* Emmaus, Pennsylvania: Rodale Press.

Taylor, Renée. 1975. *Yoga: The Art of Living.* New Canaan, Connecticut: Keats Publishing, Inc.